KEEPING JOY

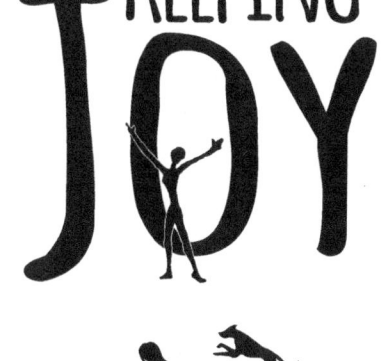

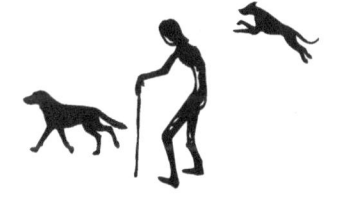

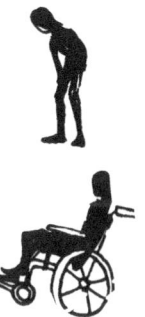

Monica-Mary
MacCallum

Published under licence by Brown Dog Books and
The Self-Publishing Partnership Ltd, 10b Greenway Farm, Bath
Rd, Wick, nr. Bath BS30 5RL

www.selfpublishingpartnership.co.uk

ISBN paperback book: 978-1-83952-565-0
ISBN e-book: 978-1-83952-566-7

Cover design by Kevin Rylands
Internal design by Andrew Easton

Printed and bound in the UK

This book is printed on FSC® certified paper

KEEPING JOY

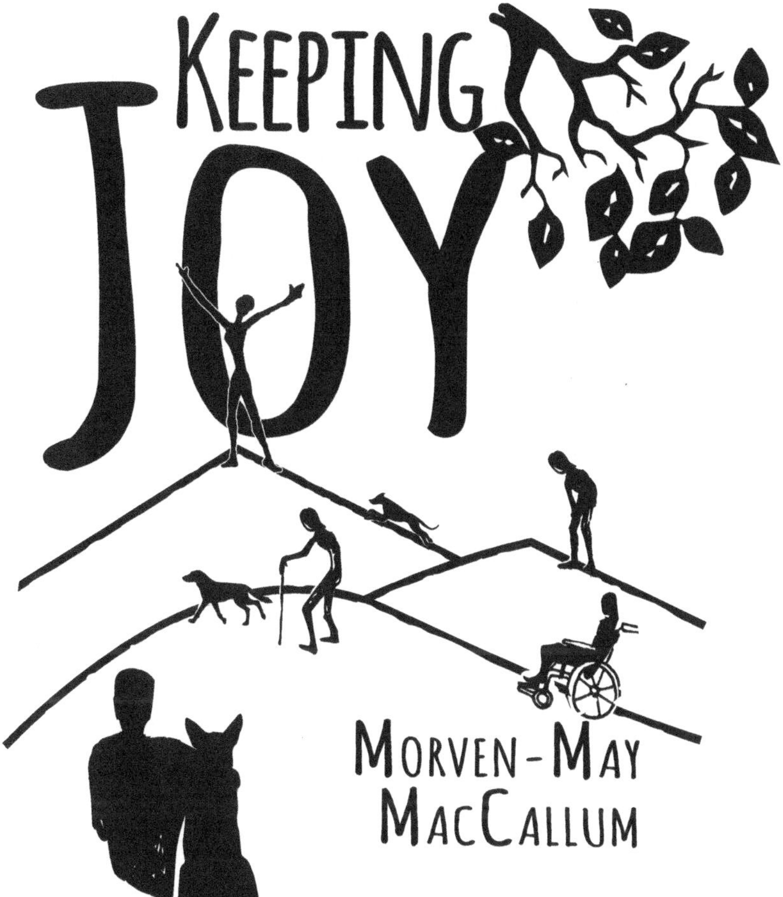

MORVEN-MAY MacCALLUM

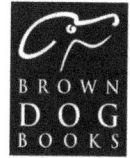

BROWN
DOG
BOOKS

I dedicate this book to you —
the constant survivor.

Chapter One

JOYCE – AGE 23

So, do you? Do you take it for granted … the simplicity of simply being able to breathe? Because I don't … I draw this secretly abused substance deep into my lungs with indulgence. And, after so many years of being trapped inside, I forever hunger to consume it.

The heat of the sun warms me until I'm glowing from the inside out – radiating something good rather than bad inside me. The glorious heat banishing the perpetual chill I'm so used to living with. I tip my head back so that the sun shines fully upon my face, the brightness turning my world into a merging shade of orange and red as the light filters through my closed eyelids. I slouch down a little on the bench, in the back garden, allowing the top slat to take the weight of my head. The peeling paint sharp against my skin. Somewhere in the distance a tractor is pacing the fields which surround my aunt's cottage, the hum of its engine a dull undertone to the chitter of the birds around me. I don't need to open my eyes to picture the mountains in the distance, the tractor nothing but a small dot in comparison. I could once have told you all the different tracks up those mountains but now I don't know if they exist.

With a sigh, I put my sunglasses back on before opening my

eyes to the world again. Despite the dark lenses, my sensitive eyes squint against the light. The peeling paint of the bench I'm meant to be refurbishing scratches at my legs as I sit up. I lean forwards in an attempt to summon up the energy to stand.

'Hi,' I whisper, reaching out my hands to Dog, who's gently padding his way towards me, my fingers instantly lost in the thickness of his fur.

Dog, my constant companion, is as big as a retriever and as hairy as a husky.

With reluctant legs, I head to the bottom of the garden, towards the shed to get some sandpaper, Dog happily following alongside me. I pull at the door, yanking at the warped wood until little by little it gives. Standing in the doorway, I pause to look about the gloomy shed, the only source of light coming from a grimy window covered in dust and cobwebs. I stare at the blurred figure of myself in the dirty glass, the auburn hair, the starkness of pale skin, my aunt's baggy old gardening coat ... I look like a fashion mannequin gone wrong. Slowly, I allow my gaze to travel from object to object. I step deeper into the shed, so that I can get a closer look at the workbench, which houses boxes of nails, brushes, sandpaper, spare parts that will probably never be used and pots of partly used paint in various colours.

I shiver in the cool air. Wrapping my arms around myself, I continue looking around ... lawnmower, tools on the wall, boxes of nails, sandpaper, boxes ... but what am I here for?

I slowly spin around on the spot, trying to work my mind.

'Come on, what was it?' I mutter.

I step towards my old mountain bike, my fingers affectionately tracing the shape of the seat and creating tracks in the dust. I spent so many hours on this thing, just Dog and I, our legs racing to outrun each other. I had to save my waitressing wage for fourteen weeks to pay for this bike. I was so proud of it and now here it lies in a dusty coffin.

I'm three chapters further into the book I'm reading when I shift my weight on the bench, the curling paint chips protruding into my bare arms abruptly reminding me of what I'm meant to be doing.

Ten minutes later, I drag the rough paper over the wooden slats of the bench, the gritty sound uncomfortable to my sensitive hearing. I ignore the pain which shoots up my wrist and forearm with each stroke and the aching in my shoulders, knees and back. My eyes, originally mesmerised by the gathering dust, are now unseeing. I just work, switching from one arm to the other when one gets too tired, my arm moving in a rhythmic motion in time to the thoughts I can't escape.

I pause to catch my breath. Assessing my work as my chest heaves under the effort my exertion is costing me. My arms hang like dead weights by my side as I straighten my back and listen to it crack like riffle fire. I still have half the bench to go and I'm spent. Four weeks ago, I did the exact same work on the table, only it was bigger and harder to sand but the effort this bench is costing is twice as much and that realisation is an uncomfortable one.

My eyes follow a lone bee as it hums past me and settles on the chaos of coloured flowers Aunt Beth asked me to plant up last week – another task which was more effort than it should have been. She was so fervent in which flowers were to go where but I think they look ridiculously ludicrous.

Dog comes over and sits beside me. His dark eyes survey me knowingly.

'I'm not getting sicker,' I tell him stubbornly, resting my

weary arm around him. He simply looks at me, his head tipped to one side and his brows raised. 'I'm not.'

I lie back on the slabs and close my eyes, allowing the warmth they've collected from the sun to leech into me, the heat within them oddly comforting.

'I'm not getting sicker,' I whisper into the sky, as the rippling in my forearm continues and as the heady weight of my body sinks deeper into the ground.

'I told you I'd finish it,' I state to Aunt Beth, two weeks later.

Trying to ignore the fact that it only took me two days to do the table – one to sand it and one to paint it.

'It looks great, you've done a good job on it,' Aunt Beth says, examining it from the kitchen window. 'Listen, I thought, seeing as I'm not working until later, that maybe we could finish decorating your room today?'

I pause, considering my rate of tiredness versus my desire to get my room finished so I can move back upstairs.

My Aunt Beth, who I've lived with since my parents died when I was seven years old and who has frequently been mistaken for my mother, was delighted when I started to show signs of wanting to decorate my old room. She makes no concealment of her desire to get her dining room back. It was converted from the dining room to my bedroom when it became blatantly clear that my illness was not the temporary inconvenience the doctors said it would be. Aunt Beth had been rightly worried about me managing the stairs when she wasn't here and she struggled to help carry me up them each night. So, the dining room was taken over by a new sofa bed. It was meant to be 'just for when I needed it' but it quickly became my permanent residence. Aunt Beth's belongings and mine continuously jostle for space as the room tries to maintain its identity.

'Yeah, I suppose so,' I say.

Aunt Beth squirms in her chair before adding, 'I had an email confirming the time for the phone consultation on Tuesday.'

'What consultation?'

'To get your blood results.'

'I thought they ... ehm ... that they came through the post?' I say with confusion, leaning against the kitchen worktop to counteract some of the aching building in my knees.

'They did ...' Aunt Beth says, a little sharply, before stopping herself and adding in a softer voice like I'm a simpleton who can't help their stupidity. 'They came through and you decided you didn't want to open them until we had a phone consultation booked – which I've booked. So, shall we open them?'

'No.' The swiftness of my reply surprises even me.

'We need to look at them, Joyce.' Aunt Beth sounds battle-worn, as though we've had this fight before.

'We may as well wait and see what Dr Hopefield says,' I tell her, unable to meet her gaze.

I don't remember deciding not to open the results, I don't remember the conversation around it and I certainly don't remember the results arriving in the first place.

'Joyce ...' Aunt Beth starts but pauses again. 'I know you don't want to go on more treatment but I know you're getting worse and that's only from what I'm seeing – so I've no idea how much worse it is given that you're the one feeling it.'

'I'm not getting licker ... sicker ... I'm getting busier. That's what you wanted – remember?' I snap, walking out of the room before Aunt Beth can reply.

The results will be fine. I am not getting sicker. I'm not.

Chapter Two

LOGAN – AGE 23

I glance over the message on the screen of my phone, inwardly cringing at it. Joy messaged a couple of days ago to tell me her test results from the private hospital … they weren't good and neither was my awkward reply of 'at least now you'll have time to watch *Men of Shadows*'. I scroll down to the last message, Joy's resounding 'thanks but not today' to my self-invitation to come over earlier making me pause … hedging my bets at how mad she'll be at me for just turning up at her house.

'Sod it,' I mutter, turning the key and waiting for the old engine to splutter into something resembling life.

I know from the bluntness of her message that she's not ok; despite her saying otherwise. It's hard to know how far to push Joy, when to leave her alone because she's not well and when to not leave her alone because she's feeling low – the two are so closely connected that it's not easy to tell them apart.

I turn right at the junction out of the farm and head down the single-track road towards her home, drumming my fingers on the steering wheel while the sun blasts down upon every surface it can touch.

I don't allow myself to pause as I turn into Joy's drive. So instead, I quickly turn off the engine, jump out the truck and head straight to the front door but, before I can get to it, Dog comes to greet me with his customary bum wiggle.

Patting his head, I take a breath before following him to the back garden – knowing that wherever Dog is, Joy will be too.

I catch sight of her sitting on a low stool, a paintbrush in hand and an open tin by her feet as she paints the bottom panel of the shed. An oversized red chequered shirt, with splatters of different colours of dried paint, adorns her body. At first, I think that's all she's wearing but as she stretches to reach further along the panel, I see she's in shorts – her pale legs almost blindingly white in the sun.

'Hey,' I say brightly, as I approach her.

'Hi,' she says, without looking round.

She must have heard me arrive, I decide; Joy's too anxious these days to not investigate any noise she's unsure of.

'… You ok?' I inwardly wince … stupid question.

'I'm fine.'

I pause, awkwardly glancing around the garden as though I'll glean inspiration from it.

'Want a cuppa?' I ask, sounding like my mother.

'I just want to get this done before …'

'… Ok,' I say quietly.

After a moment of hesitation, I head into the shed and rummage around until I find a paintbrush which has definitely seen better days. I crouch down beside her and dip my scruffy brush in the tin and start to paint. Joy pauses to watch me. I try to pretend I don't notice. I try to act like this is completely natural, a prearranged event, but nothing feels normal … even the brush in my hand feels alien. I'm about to dip my brush in the paint again when Joy gets to her feet and slowly disappears into the cottage.

I pause, my insides sinking. I should have known not to come. I'm about to get up and leave, with some excuse about helping my dad on the farm, when she reappears with another chequered shirt and hands it to me.

'… Thanks,' I say, pulling the shirt on over my t-shirt. 'I don't think your red one would have brought out my eyes.'

I glance at her, as I say it, to see her lips pulling together as though to resist a smile and then she finally looks at me, her eyes mingled with so many emotions it's hard to discern them all; sadness, pain, humour, but I think what I see most clearly is gratitude.

'Suits you,' she says meekly, tucking a clump of her dark auburn hair behind her ears.

'You think?' I say, grabbing the corners of the shirt and pulling them out from my skin like a skirt.

'You're an idiot,' she scoffs but with a small smile.

I shrug and pick up my brush again – I don't mind looking like an idiot if it makes her smile.

Joy works quietly, methodically, going over all the bits I've missed, trying all the while not to make it obvious that she's doing so but within twenty minutes I'm beyond bored.

'Tea break,' I order, getting up and heading into the cottage. 'Human tea or rabbit tea?'

'Ehh,' Joy ponders, looking at her work, as though comparing the effort against what beverage she deserves in exchange. 'Human tea.'

I nod and head inside, navigating the small kitchen with the familiarity of someone who's more than just a guest despite not being an inhabitant.

I snatch glances of Joy through the kitchen window as I make us a cup each. It's hard to think that within a few weeks or so that she'll start treatment, and go back to being that bedbound shadow that she fought so hard to be free from. I rub my ribs as I wait for the kettle to boil, feeling like the strike of her news has ricocheted off her and hit me too, as though I have a dulled version of the wound she's just been blown. I honestly don't know how she's still standing.

When I step outside, juggling two overfull mugs, she's already sitting on the bench waiting for me.

'So ... how are you?' I ask, handing her a mug. 'And don't say fine,' I cut her off as the words form on her lips.

She sighs.

'Say it. Whatever it is, you can say it.'

She shrugs one shoulder and looks down at the mug cradled in her hands. 'I don't know what you want me to say.'

'You must be angry,' I hedge, thinking of how I feel on her behalf.

She exhales a short breath from her nose and tilts her head slightly in a way that lets me know that I've said something stupid.

'Spit it out,' I nudge her gently.

She pauses, as though thinking of how to say what she wants to express. 'I am angry somewhere, it's just exhausting to feel it and I can't do anything with it ... I can't get it out of me so what's the point ... I'm more worried about the day when I am well enough to feel it.'

'... Maybe you need to find little outlets for it, every now and then, so it doesn't build up,' I suggest.

'Like what? I can hardly go for a run ... I tried that – remember.'

I grimace, unable to stop the memory of sitting by her hospital bedside for hours on end after she attempted, I suppose she also succeeded, to prove the public doctors wrong about her illness not being in her head ... not that it helped. They still wouldn't treat her but it set Aunt Beth on the trail to get her private treatment.

'Yeah, not your best move,' I say, my voice muffled as I bring my mug up to my lips to take a sip.

We lapse into silence, Dog panting by our feet.

'That shed is a disgusting colour by the way,' I observe, glaring at the vile brown shade like faded muck which is slowly drying in the sun.

'At least you don't have to look at it,' she retorts.

'I do when I visit,' I mutter.

'Yeah, well, you'll be back at uni soon. Besides, shouldn't you be with your family?' she remarks, sipping her tea.

'Just wanted to check in,' I say, gently.

We fall back into silence but my mind is whirring.

'Back in a minute,' I say decisively, downing the last of my tea and handing her the empty mug.

I race back to the truck and, even though there's no need to rush, I hastily open the passenger door and rummage inside my rucksack. Locating what I'm hunting for, I sprint back to Joy. I throw her the boxes I've taken from my bag and wait for her reaction as she examines them.

'Condoms ... really? I appreciate the offer but I think that would be crossing a boundary. Also, why have you got so ... ehh ...'

'Many?' I venture. 'We were going to prank my brother for his birthday but it never really happened so ...' I point to the shed.

'I don't think that would be comfortable,' she says dubiously.

'What ... no. Paint bombs,' I say proudly.

'Are you serious?'

'Yup, gets your anger out, makes the shed colourful, uses up all those tins you have in there, which, by the way, I remember being there when we were in school and we can always paint it over so Aunt Beth won't go mental.'

I can feel the anticipation in my muscles … preparing to duck the condom boxes which I'm certain she's about to throw at me. A part of me even hopes she does, just so I can see a little glimmer of the Joy she once was.

'I'll get a funnel,' she says instead.

'Put some effort into it,' Joy mocks, ten minutes later, throwing a paint-filled condom at the shed.

I watch as it hits the wooden frame, the condom stretching like dough before bursting, to splatter peach paint on the shed walls.

'I didn't think they'd be so robust,' I say defensively, taking aim and hurling the slimy condom which once again hits the shed, bounces off and lands pathetically on the grass.

'You clearly got all the ones from the cheap box,' I try to justify, striding off to collect my unbroken condom bomb, as Joy's burst bright pink upon impact.

'Put your anger into it,' Joy says as I return, mimicking my earlier words back to me.

After a few more failed attempts, I get the knack for getting the bombs to burst and before long the shed is a multicoloured rainbow that would have put Joseph's jacket to shame.

'Last two,' Joy says a little breathlessly, her arms lagging as she tries to pass me one. Her hand falling too far to the left and then the right as she tries and fails to locate my hand.

'Ready,' I say, taking it from her instead and trying to ignore what I've seen. 'Three, two … one.'

We hurl the bombs with all we have and watch as they land just under the newspaper-covered window, the paint slowly running down the wall to merge with the other colours.

'We should sign it,' she suggests.

'Mhhh … I'm not sure I want your Aunt Beth to have evidence of my involvement in this.'

'So, did that get any of your anger out?' I ask, nodding towards the shed twenty minutes later as we sit on the patio with a rabbit tea each.

'I think I got something better out of it instead,' she says with a small smile but her words are sombre, her moment of joy somehow filling her with sadness.

'I don't know what to do,' she says abruptly.

'About your treatment?' I hedge.

'Yeah,' she says, running her fingers along the sandy grout of the slabs.

'I guess … I guess, you do whatever you need to do to get the best life that you can have,' I tell her.

She stares at me like I've been replaced with a stranger.

'I know,' I say in surprise. 'I've no idea where that came from either.'

She smiles a little and shakes her head in disbelief. 'How do you do that, though, when you don't know what either of the outcomes will be? The treatment will make me so much worse but so will staying off it … the only difference is the time frame,' she explains, as plainly as if she were giving a weather update. 'Sorry,' she says stoically, her hand once more tracing the slabs.

'Everything will be ok,' I say as brightly as I can, putting my arm around her and pulling her to me.

I feel her warmth against me and silently sigh, wishing that my words were convincing enough to fool us.

Chapter Three

BETH

Count to three, this life is for me. One, I'm numb. Two, I've gone dumb. Three, I can't stop thinking. Count to three, there's still more to see. One, where've you gone. Two, I know what you've done. Three, is for overthinking. Count to three, this life is for me …

I repeat the words over and over again, trying in vain to remember the rest of the rhyme. I used to say it to myself when my husband and I got divorced. I never understood how dark the other side of him could be until then … I never knew I had a darker side myself.

I slowly take a sip from my cup, allowing my eyes to survey the perfectly manicured garden of my customer's home. I finished work ten minutes ago but the lady who owns this fine Victorian house insisted on making me something to drink before I left; so, I asked if I could take it in the garden and she seemed pleased by my suggestion to do so. I follow the gravel path, enjoying the gentle crunch the expensively fine gravel makes underneath my feet. I think of my partly tarred (which was already there when we bought the ground) and ugly bog-standard stones back home; which have been down so long they're now compacted solidly into the tracks my tyres make.

I can't help but make a mental note of all the things I want one day and of all the things I don't. In my fantasy world, I don't have a sick niece who was misdiagnosed for years, while the illness inside her devoured her physical and mental strength. I don't have a house I had to re-mortgage to pay for the private treatment to keep her from dying. I don't go home each night exhausted after working every hour that's given to me as an electrician.

In my fantasy, Joyce's illness would be diagnosed and treated early and, as it should have been, she would have recovered within six weeks. She'd even have graduated from university by now. And me, well, I wouldn't have had to watch my sister's daughter almost die under my care. In my fantasy, I get to live a life that's lived for me and not for her.

I pause to take a sip as I admire the neatly cut hedges, the expert lines of the borders and the flowers so pleasantly arranged within it … and then I think of my weed-ridden, overgrown, colourless, unmanageable and untameable jungle back home; which isn't even half the size of this woman's perfect garden.

I shouldn't complain. Joyce spent ages carefully planting up the flower boxes, which had still contained the corpses of the flowers from the previous year, I didn't have the heart to pull them up to coordinate them so that the colours didn't clash. It's my own fault. I should have put the flowers that were for the back garden round the back for her, instead of telling her which ones were for the back and which were for the front – I should have known that these days she'd get them confused. But I underestimated just how sick she's become again … I think I still do.

I follow the path around a tight bend and through an archway in the hedge. I pause underneath it to take in the beautiful pond.

The still expanse of water disturbed by the gentle trickle of a water feature, of a man and a woman, towards the bottom end of the pond. The stone figures are holding an umbrella each, their other arms linked … they look as though they're dancing in the rain, with such unbridled happiness that it's hard to take your eyes off them.

I wonder if the pond's deep enough to swim in or if the little wooden pier is just for show. Either way, I walk to the end of it. I ease my weary body down upon the wooden slats so that I'm sitting with my legs dangling off the end – the tips of my boots just touching the water. It's so peaceful it's perturbing. This woman's home, her garden, it's everything mine used to be to me. The cottage was never a grand house but to me it was my castle. My husband and I built it brick by brick, pipe by pipe, wire by wire. I never foresaw, within those beautifully restored windows, that I would go from being a wife and a mother of one; to being a divorced, single mother of three.

I sigh deeply before drinking my last mouthful of tea, watching as the heel of my tattered boot lightly touches the top of the water. Tentatively, I submerge my foot a little more as though testing to see how deep I can sink – before the cold water infiltrates my boot.

Slowly, I stretch out my fingers, the warmth from the cup no longer subduing the aching in them now its empty.

I watch my fingers flex and contract around the chilled china, remembering how cold Joyce was the night she came to me. I was engrossed in a hill of paperwork, so much so that I didn't even notice her enter the room.

'Aunt Beth,' she said in such a small voice that, when I looked up, I half expected to see the seven-year-old version of her.

She was perched on the arm of the couch, neither dedicated to staying nor fully committed to leaving. She was hunched over, one arm clutched in the other.

'I need to go back to the hospital.'

And with that she broke down, as though her denial had been the only thing holding her together. I paused, so taken aback by her admission that I was frozen in time, a pen in one hand and a handful of paperwork in the other.

'You don't need to go back, you're doing really well.'

'I'm not, it's back,' she insisted beseechingly, holding out her arm as though it were some kind of clue.

I got up and stood beside her. Putting an arm around her, I said, 'You're just tired.'

'I'm not, it's back, I can feel it inside me. It's attacking me. My arm's been numb for days and now it won't stop tingling and twitching,' she said imploringly.

I looked down at the arm she was cradling and watched as her thumb and the last two digits on her hand jerked and danced to a rhythm which was not of her making. That's when I started to pay attention and that's when I saw how much of her this disease had already reclaimed.

I shake my head. I can't stand to remember any more. I make myself get to my feet and head back to my customer's home. I leave a note in the room I was working in, under the china mug, to say thanks and how much I enjoyed her garden.

I'm so used to Joyce being in bed when I get home from work that I do a double take when I walk through the back door to find her preparing dinner.

I call out a greeting as I hang my coat in the utility room

and then take a seat in the kitchen. I pretend to update my calendar for work while sneaking glances of assessment at her. She's stooping more and more these days come evening time, like the sped-up progression of old age, all within one day, her body slowly shrinking, wizening and weakening. Her gait, as she moves around the kitchen, is short; her feeble feet hardly leaving the ground as she slowly shuffles from one place to the other – her closest hand holding onto the counter top to support her. I wonder if she sees her regression, she surely must feel the pain of it, or is she so determined to keep putting one foot in front of the other that her focus blinds her?

I watch as she tests if the potatoes are cooked before lifting the pan. My hands shooting to the edge of the table, preparing to push myself up, as her arms tremble so violently that boiling water slops over the rim of the pan and sizzles on the heat of the ring. She half drops, half places, the pan back down before opening a drawer and taking out a slotted spoon to drain the few potatoes she's boiled.

I look away, unable to watch. I quickly get up from the table and hasten to collect some cutlery from the drawers. 'I thought we could eat outside,' I say.

I don't look at her as I shut the drawer and head outside before she can answer me. I flinch as the back door bangs behind me – knowing how much the noise will make Joyce jump from her hyper-sensitive hearing. I clutch my handful of cutlery to my chest, as though the tighter I hold the cold metal the more I can prevent the compressing of my heart. Slowly, I let my head fall back against the door as I release the breath I've been holding. It gushes out of me in a shuddering exhumation of despair.

How could I have ever believed that monster was gone, that

our lives could only go up from here because, surely, how much worse could they have gotten ... how unbelievably naïve I've been, how stupid. I remember all the terse retorts Joyce would say whenever I uttered such notions ... she knew all along she'd never be free of it. I take a few shuddering breaths until they even out. I don't have time to break down, I remind myself. I don't have time to break. I have no choice but to be strong because I'm afraid that if I let myself fall apart, then I'll never find a way to put myself back together.

I lift my head, sniff at my running nose and step away from the back door to set the table on the patio ... instead, I'm struck still as I'm confronted by the multicoloured monstrosity which was previously my shed. With the cutlery forgotten in my hand, I walk towards it and stare at it in utter dismay. Slowly, my eyes start to pick out the more random splodges of colour splattered all over it, the merging of the various colours as they run into one another.

'I can paint over it,' comes Joyce's feeble voice from behind me.

I slowly turn around to face her. She looks even more shrunken than she did five minutes ago, as though the effort of just being has stolen even more of her height.

'Actually ... I like it,' I tell her, taking the few steps necessary to stand beside her on the patio to stare at it. 'I always said I wanted colour in the garden.'

'Really?' she asks sceptically, I simply nod.

'Mh hm, it's very ... original,' I say, before heading inside to get our plates.

'Have you decided what you're going to do?' I ask, a few minutes later, trying to casually cut my potato as though the answer contains no consequences.

She shrugs half-heartedly, moving her food across her plate rather than eating it.

I watch her. I'm trying my best but it's hard, when someone's so dependent on you, to not dictate their lives for them. It makes life so much easier to just decide on her behalf; in the desire for an easier life, I don't even notice half the time that I'm taking away hers. I still can't bring myself to tell her that I opened her results before the phone consultation. I paid for them and besides, I reason, I needed to know what they said in order to do my research so that I could ask the relevant questions.

'If you don't want to do it … you don't have to,' I manage to tell her despite the ache in my throat.

'This will be my third round of treatment.'

'I know,' I say softly.

'I don't know if I can do it again,' Joyce mutters morosely, looking down at her plate.

'It's only three months,' I remind her, chewing on a bit of dried-out chicken.

'It's not just three months. It's the six months of recovering and rebuilding all the ground I've gained since the last treatment.'

'I know,' I say dejectedly. A heavy silence falling before us and I'm glad of the birds whose evening calls fill the air between us.

'Just think of all the things you can do now which you couldn't do before you started all this treatment. Think of how much more you'll be able to do after you've recovered this round.'

'Is it worth it?'

I hesitate, unsure if it's a rhetorical question or not.

I study her pale face, the paint flecks in her auburn hair, the eyes which move to stare into a place I can't reach. I bite the inside of my mouth, my heart physically aching, I see so much of my sister within her. I tuck a strand of her hair behind her ear and for a moment all the stress and all the worry of how I'll pay for this falls away.

'Of course, it is.'

Her eyes flick toward me but she doesn't meet my gaze because we both know her spells of improvement are so fleeting in comparison to their cost.

We eat the rest of our dinner mostly in silence, pausing occasionally to comment on the freshly decorated shed and Logan's creative influence upon it, as the evening sun weakens its hold in the sky ... there really is no escaping the approaching darkness.

Chapter Four

JOYCE – AGE 23

THE IRONY OF ILLNESS:
- Furniture – Bedside table or mini pharmacy?
- Multitasking – The washing's in the dishwasher, the dishes are in the washing machine, the dinner's in the dryer and the clothes are in the oven … I got this down!
- Sleep – I eventually got the recommended eight hours of sleep! It took me eleven days but it still counts, doesn't it?
- Memory – I know I have a bad memory but a lot of the time I don't remember …

I lie on my back, listening to the ticking of my bedside clock. It's meant to be silent but it's as temperamental as my teetering health. It's garishly large, meant for the elderly I suspect, with its oversized numbers and oversized snooze button – which I pound with a weak vengeance whenever it goes off.

When I was on treatment, the ticking of my old clock ignited my tinnitus and the two sets of ticking at different times and pitches, on top of my baseline hum, drove me to distraction … hummm, tick, TICK, tick, hummm TICK, tick, hummm. So, I've forgiven this giant clock for its bouts of sound in exchange for the relief its silence brings me.

It's been well over a week since I got the results from the private hospital and, every morning since, I've played a game of will I or won't I. Ten more ticks and I *will* get out of bed, I tell myself in preparation. Three. Two. One … my body is unmoving. The *won't* is always more seductive than the *will*. Ok, I order myself, actually get up this time! Three. Two. One … I heave myself upright and drag my legs out of my sofa bed in preparation to stand. I sit for a moment, my head swimming, groggy and unfocused. I haul myself upright and step towards the end of my bed, but as I put my weight onto my left leg, my entire body lurches in that direction. Vaguely, I feel the floor compressing the soft flesh of my foot but there's no sensation, no balance, no way to tell where to put my weight to counter myself as I careen to one side. My right leg staggers forward to counteract but instead it propels me forwards towards the floor. I hear before I feel the solid thump of my head hitting off the floor and the gasp of pain it induces a second later.

I lie still … too scared to move, glitter popping before my eyes like a poor party popper.

'It's ok, it's ok,' I whisper to myself, my ragged breath catching in my throat.

Slowly, I reach round for the metal legs of my sofa bed, the cold metal clutched in my hands like the rope of a life raft, as I use the frame of the bed and my good leg to haul myself across the floor, my left leg dragging behind me like a fresh corpse. I pull myself upright before shuffling myself, a little bit at a time, until I can lean my back against the frame. I stare at my left leg, my hand hovering over it, but I can't bring myself to touch it.

Slowly, with a shaking hand, I reluctantly reach down to touch my leg. I release a guttural breath – I can't feel my fingers

… I can't even feel the movement of them on my skin. With desperation, I dig my fingers into my leg until the skin goes deathly white and the imprint of my nails is gouged into my flesh like a temporary tattoo … but all I can feel is a dull sensation of the impression of something on my leg. I take a breath and then hit my leg as hard as I can, the palm and the pads of my hand smarting with the impact, but my leg feels nothing.

With trepidation, I try wiggling my toes but the connection feels severed.

'No …' I plead silently, wrapping my arms around my aching lungs – neither of them fully able to expel or inhale the air I require from them.

I try again and again to move my toes. It's a conscious effort but, after a moment, they do move … even if I can't feel it, they do move.

I run my hands over my leg, back and forth, faster and faster. Trying to encourage blood flow; even though I've no idea if that's the cause of my numbness. It doesn't help … I hit my leg, over and over again until my arms feel like lead and are too tired to continue my own self-beating. I want to get up but I'm frightened too. Instead, I pull the duvet off the bed and lie there, the stillness my only companion. It could be worse, I tell myself. It could be worse …

My chest is heaving. I know it must be, because surely my heart's pounding. I know my body is where I left it last night, safe and warm inside my sofa bed, but that's all I feel … there's nothing else. I try to move my pinkie, that slim stick of bones, but nothing happens. I try to open my eyes, to sit up. I feel as though my innards might be pushing upwards or maybe it's the residual memory of the motion but, either way, I'm not moving – nothing is moving. I frantically order my brain to command my body to move. I try to think through the process of the act but still I'm trapped. I can think, I can feel I have a body attached to my brain but everything else is gone. The connection severed ... I'm paralysed.

I don't know how long I lie there for but slowly the first pinpricks of pain start shooting through my leg like fireworks popping into hundreds of tiny bursts of maleficent sparks – until my leg is covered in a thousand burns. I fight the urge to clench my teeth against the pain, my breathing shallow as I tell myself that it's only as painful as I let it be ... but that's a lie. It bloody hurts. I can't tell how long it takes but finally the sensation in my leg slowly returns and with it the passing of the pain, but there are random patches of numbness; especially on my thigh.

I get up slowly, carefully testing my leg before I dare to put my weight on it. Mistrusting myself. Once I'm sure my legs can hold me, I make my way to the kitchen using the walls for stability.

Dog is waiting for me in the kitchen. His head tilted to one side, his tail flicking slowly back and forth, his big endearing eyes holding mine; like he knows what's happened and is telling me I'm ok. But I don't feel ok. How can any of this be ok?

I pull out the nearest of the kitchen chairs and sink my body onto it, leaning forwards until I'm bent double, I open my arms as I hear Dog's claws gently clipping against the tiled floor. His head nuzzles into my shoulder as I wrap my arms around him in a hug. I fight back tears which nonetheless soak his coat. I don't know what I'm more afraid of – going onto treatment or staying off it.

Five days later, I sit on the floor of my bedroom with my legs crossed beneath me, like we were made to sit during primary school, with Dog lying beside me. My eyes tracing the swirling pattern of the new sage green wallpaper on the back wall. I purse my lips, still unsure if I like the changes I've made – it's hard to know what you like when who you are has been stolen from you. I glance around me, aware that somehow the room feels warped, as though it's now no longer fully the old me but nor has it developed into the representation of the person I was becoming – its creation, like mine, has been halted before it could form.

We finished decorating a while ago but it's taken until now for me to start clearing away all the bits of off-cut wallpaper, the pasting table and brushes. I've spent most of the afternoon manically putting the room back together. I don't really know why I was so frantic in my efforts to get the room sorted – perhaps it was the arrival of the ominously large box of drugs at lunchtime which evoked the notion.

I think I wanted to be able to shut the door on what this room began to represent. I want to be able to lock away the person I was becoming and retreat back into the person I was before I started to believe that I could be something more than sick … that person from before knows how to survive what I'm about to endure … this new one doesn't.

Yet despite the complete transformation of the walls being painted cream, and wallpaper where there was never any before, of new curtains and matching bedsheets … I still can't shake the ghost of Joy.

No matter what I do I can't expel the phantom of the old me from this place. It's as though she haunts this room more than me or any other part of the cottage and no matter what I do, this room is keeping Joy … I only wish I'd known how to keep her too. I can still see myself, the teenage Joy and her friends sitting in a circle on my bedroom floor, laughing and joking and planning our next adventure out camping, or of us coming home after an eight-hour cycle, our muddy and scratched legs a testament to our adventures. But she's gone and so are the friends who abandoned her.

I close my eyes and let my memories take me to a world where I was the closest to happiness that I've ever been. They comfort me and haunt me all at the same time because the person I was is so far removed from who I am – that it seems impossible for her to have ever been me. I can see my Joy sitting at the desk studying for upcoming exams. I can see her racing to get up and out the door each morning for her 5am run with Dog. These memories play before my closed eyes like a moving scene in a film. A life so big it seems impossible that it could ever have been contained within this room.

Sometimes I wander from room to room as though if I retrace my steps, I might find myself, but all I find are ghosts.

This was the life I had deluded myself into believing I could get back.

The shadows of Joy were there, I could see them growing stronger as I did, waiting for me to embody them once more but there is no denying it now. There is no illusion left to delude myself with. The results are in, the drugs have arrived, my time in dreamland is up, my reprieve retracted. I am re-entering the world of the sick rather than the recovering.

I accepted it that morning I collapsed on the floor with a deadened leg. I messaged Aunt Beth that very afternoon and asked her to order the medication.

My hands grip tightly onto the outsides of my thighs. I'm meant to start treatment in a few days. I know what the private hospital and my aunt want me to do and I know I said I'd do it but I'm not sure I can. I'm not sure I want to. I close my eyes, wrapping my arms around my waist as my insides sink further than I ever thought it possible for them to fall, tears falling silently down my cheeks. My tissue stinging for the chill piercing my body. I don't understand how this has become my life.

I sigh heavily and open my eyes, glad to be alone. Aunt Beth seemed glad too to be called to an emergency homer on her only day off. I'm better alone anyway, I tell myself. I've been housebound for six years now and a lot of that was spent being bedbound. I've survived this far. I can feel the corners of my mouth drooping downwards, like there's invisible buckets upon the ends which are slowly collecting my tears, the weight of my sorrow pulling them downwards with every tear they catch.

My hand automatically reaches for Dog. I'm not even aware of my fingers moving through his coat until they lock in place, hovering over a lump on his neck. I sit up, rigid and alert. I carefully draw the hair over the lump apart to see a tiny but still engorged black-bodied tick buried in Dog's skin. As quickly as my cumbersome body allows me, I get myself up off the floor, my knees cracking sharply.

'Stay,' I order, when Dog looks like he's about to move.

I go downstairs to the kitchen and find the tick remover before grabbing a sheet of kitchen roll. I drag my weak and unwilling legs up the stairs and head back to my room. I ease the two-pronged fork under the legs of the tick and twirl it round, being careful not to pull it, until the stubborn beast finally comes away cleanly with the head still attached. I hold it up to eye level. The tiny monster with a head so small I can hardly see it, trapped in the remover, its eight spindly legs kicking out like a toddler mid-tantrum. I wonder if this one contains it; the bacteria which reduced me from a teenager full of life ... into the stunted thing I am today.

I marvel at how something so small could have something so powerful within it. I heard Aunt Beth say the spirochete, which is the Lyme disease bacteria, is thinner than a strand of hair.

Even though I'm evidence of it, it still seems impossible to me that something so commonplace, so seemingly insignificant as a tick bite could leave you fighting for your life. Even now, even after battling for years with the public health system, I still can't comprehend the medical ignorance around it, the lack of reliable testing, the sheer number of people who are misdiagnosed and refused treatment because of that and how many people, just like me, who are left to fend for themselves or die trying. All thanks to a tiny tick and what it might carry. It fascinates me and nauseates me all at the same time.

I wrap the tick in kitchen roll and slowly make my way back downstairs. At the back door I pick up a rock and, making sure it's well wrapped in the paper, I press the rock as hard as I can on top of the tick before taking it inside and putting it inside the wood burner – watching as the blackness spreads across the white paper before it bursts into flames. You'd think I would feel fear, holding the soldier of my enemy ... but I feel nothing and nor is there satisfaction in watching it burn.

Chapter Five

JOYCE – AGE 23

Round one of treatment was torture … I think we can all agree on that. Round two was equally as unpleasant … only it came with the added burden of knowing what would come. Round three is … all of the above but the fact that it's round three just makes it sheer cruelty.

Today's the day, the first day of regression in the hope of progression. The drugs which are so commonplace that people think they contain no consequences for consuming them sit in my trembling hand; whether I tremble from fear or from the Lyme itself, I don't know. I can't bring myself to ingest them though, to place the poison that will help to heal me into my mouth. They sit on my palm for so long that they begin to stick to my skin. When I finally bring myself to do it, with a swift movement followed by a mouthful of water, I find my reluctance is not only emotional but physical. It comes from my very body, which refuses to swallow the pills floating against the roof of my mouth. It's like my body knows what will happen and it knows it can't endure any more. It's only as the capsules begin to dissolve and I can start to taste the rancidness of them that I finally manage to swallow them down in one … painful … gulp.

I grab at the edges of the kitchen worktop, the glass in my hand almost falling to the floor as I hasten to put it down, images flashing before my eyes like my own personalised horror story. Memories of things I thought I'd forgotten blind my sight. They come at me like hologram images, only stronger, physically felt, smelt and tasted as well as seen. I sink to the stone floor, my knees giving out from under me. I clutch at my heaving ribs as a strangled cry emanates from within me.

I can't breathe.

I gasp snatches of air through the pain as an image of myself, reflected in the bathroom mirror, stares back at me ... I'm skeletal, my lips blue, eyes dark like the light's been sucked from them, sunken and almost swollen shut, my face the pallor of death. I hold onto my ribs, knowing that they're now covered in flesh but still somehow feeling the bones as sharply as if they had nothing to cover them but skin. I drag another breath into my lungs, feeling the cold roughness of the bathroom floor as I drag myself across it until I can go no further, drenched in sweat but too weak to even shiver out the chill which pierces my body like barbed wire. I can smell the vile stench of sickness that oozes from my pores and infects my room and the taste of decay in my mouth as my insides are poisoned and begin to rot. I order myself to stop, to cut it out, but it keeps on coming. My head aches agonisingly from pain I know isn't there yet and my face tingles from air I can't consume. I want to be sick, to hurl the tablets I've taken into me back out. It takes everything I have not to.

'I can't do this,' I mouth, my voice so strangled that there's no sound.

I dig my nails into my flesh until I'm sure my skin will burst but I stop myself ... scared of what my blood contains. As soon as

I can, I haul myself off the floor and stagger to my dining room – the world around me disorientating. It only takes half an hour to feel the drugs start to strangle my strength, the heavy weight of my body carried under shaking limbs whose muscles are rendered redundant.

When I was a child, before my parents died, I would have this dream where I was a bird. This beautiful, colourful bird who sang so loudly and soared so high through the blue sky. Then, out of nowhere, I'd be spiralling downwards in a dizzying whirlwind of nothingness. Often, I woke before I hit the ground but sometimes … sometimes I didn't and when I got up off the ground, stunned and dazed I'd find myself caged, in a darkened room, locked behind bars. I never saw my captor, who loomed at me from the shadows but, as the days stretched on, I lost my voice, my feathers fell, my extremities became too exhausted to even try to fly, I began to die and I welcomed it. When I woke up, tears on my chubby child cheeks, I would think how lucky I was that that would never be me.

'Joyce, are you awake?' Aunt Beth whispers into the darkened dining room, two months into my treatment.

I open my mouth to reply but I can't remember how. I try desperately to speak. To make a sound as the strip of light, coming through my open door, slowly disappears as my aunt shuts the door behind her and I'm plunged back into darkness. I gasp in a ragged breath. I know there's air in my lungs but I feel breathless … suffocated. There's never enough air. I slowly curl into a tight ball, the pain inside me momentarily easing before resurging. The ice oozing from my frozen fingers spreading into my skin wherever my fingers meet what little warmth's still left in my flesh. There is nothing left but the cold and the darkness and I am its vessel.

I sweat despite the ice inside me. The pain raking through my body like the claws of a vicious monster, which loves to leave me lying at the feet of death.

'Joyce?' Aunt Beth says again, coming back into my room.

I struggle to open my eyes, unsure if this is the same day ... or a new one?

Aunt Beth walks around my sofa bed and turns on the light. I flinch fractionally, my eyes burning against the soft light of the lamp. My eyes so swollen from exhaustion that I can barely see. I try to speak but I ... I can't remember ... I can't ... I.

'It's ok,' Aunt Beth says softly. 'Take your time.'

Routine reminds me that I know what this means and this time there is no stopping the beseeching whimper which emanates from my emaciated core. No, please no, please just stop, my body begs. But it never ends and it never stops and for some reason neither do I. My body shudders as I try to push myself upright, my arms trembling with weakness. These feeble, fragile things ... how strong they are to bear the weight they're burdened with. Aunt Beth helps me to sit up, my back cracking and popping like wet wood in a fire, loud, sharp and reverberating. My chest heaves, breathless with the effort of existing. I feel rather than see my aunt sit down on my sofa bed. I try to open my eyes wider but the light burns them. I slowly turn my head towards the lamp, hoping against hope that Aunt Beth will notice and, after a moment, she does.

'Is it too bright?' she asks softly.

I nod once ... it's all I can manage for the searing burning in my neck. Aunt Beth leans forward and the snap of the switch as she turns it off reverberates agonisingly through my ears and into the core of my brain, but at least the pressure behind my eyes and in my mind has stopped.

Aunt Beth, her slim frame fuller than it used to be, roughly scrapes back her dark hair – preparing for her mission in the glow of the near soundless TV. She begins to spoon-feed me my dinner and, as the cold metal and the warm mashed potato enters my mouth, my sluggish brain seems to recognise this as the first human contact I've had all day.

The serpent of nausea hisses as it starts coiling and uncoiling inside my stomach. Halfway through, Aunt Beth pauses to spoon a handful of tablets into my mouth. She holds up a glass with a straw in it for me to drink from; as I attempt to swallow them. She then continues to feed me my dinner – layering my stomach both bottom and top against the damage the meds could do to its lining. But still, I feel the impact of every tablet as it lands and dissolves in my stomach, the explosion which ripples out like shockwaves, sending my innards reeling as the vile taste of them seeps up through my gums and makes my brain ache.

I'm a good patient though, an obedient child; I haven't the mental or physical ability to be anything otherwise. I swallow the food which I'm too tired to chew. I try not to choke as shockwaves of pain mingle with the aching in my jaw from my futile attempts to eat with civility. In return, my Aunt Beth cooks soft foods and sits with patience as I catch my breath from the exertion this sustenance inflicts upon me. I say my please and thank yous, when I can remember how to, as she half carries me to the bathroom and sits me on the toilet and waits for me to finish. She tries her best not to degrade me as she helps to pull my pyjama bottoms up around me and, in return, I try my best not to let her see me cry. She gently brushes my yellowed and now loose-fitting teeth and I, in turn, try not to beg her not to: terrified my teeth will fall out the way my auburn hair has fallen and thinned like a threadbare rug.

And all the while the vicious voice whispers in the darkness … what's the point?

'Joyce, you're so close to the end of your treatment – why don't you stop? A week or so won't make any difference?' Aunt Beth asks beseechingly, as she has done each night for … I don't really remember.

I know the days change but her reasonings never do. I remember her sitting as she is now, through two previous rounds of treatment, begging me to stop – she's scared the treatment will kill me; I'm scared it won't.

I ignore her. I know I have a reason not to stop but thoughts fail me. Pain encases me. My body disintegrates before me. I look at the long fingers of the hand on my knee and I don't know who they belong to. I think they're mine but they're too old to be. No, they're the woman's. I don't know where she came from or why she sits so sadly on my bed, her back hunched in defeat and her face pinched by sorrow's fingers.

'Ok,' she says disparagingly. I don't know what I've done to disappoint her. 'Come on, last mouthful,' she says so kindly that I don't refuse, not wanting to sadden her further. I open my hanging mouth as wide as the stiffness in my jaw will allow … I am an obedient child.

The lady leaves the room and an involuntary shudder of pain seizes me with more. The food I've ingested sits so heavily that surely it must tear through the lining of my stomach. I can feel all my organs straining to function as one. I can sense everything within me that's under attack; the blood in my veins which feels like acid, the marrow in my bones devoured by the boreholes of this bacteria, the tissue swelling with the poison released by the dying of this disease, my habitually pounding heart, which frequently and frighteningly misses a beat; my brain … my beautiful brain no longer contains thought.

Thoughtlessness is a mercy. It mutes the thoughts of death's debate. The sound of the TV is nothing but jumbled noise, my brain too slow to break apart each word that's said or to understand its meaning, my eyes too tired and sluggish to follow the characters on the screen. I slowly look around the darkened room. Just trying to make my eyes move requires focus – I feel their every movement within their sockets, the weight of my eyeballs inside my skull. I feel death's presence beside me, keeping me company while teasing me with its refusal to grant me mercy. I lie there, day in and day out. The effort it takes to expand my chest to breathe is astounding. The pain, the burning, searing, aching, knowing, shooting, biting pain … is more than I can ask my body to bear.

My skeletal frame is so fragile that the woman doesn't dare touch it unless she has to. I sleep but I don't expect to wake. I cry although I don't know why. I feel nothing, even my soul seems to have sought safety in desertion. There is no such thing as time or substance and everything is unmeasurable. I am a living corpse … rotting from the inside out. I can taste it, I can smell it, my own body decaying from the inside out.

Chapter Six

BETH

I silently go through my mental list of things I need to do for Joyce before tomorrow and tick them off on my fingers until I run out of fingers to count on.

- Her breakfast – ready to be heated in the morning and left in the thermal bowl for when she wakes.
- Her lunch – made and in the cool bag.
- A flask of tea – ready for making up in the morning.
- Bottles of water with lemon – in the fridge ready to leave in her room to ensure she's drinking enough (the lemon helps with detoxing – it's a small but powerful thing).
- A little box of nuts for snacking on – even though she never eats them.
- Leave the kettle only a quarter full – in the near non-existent chance she might try to lift it.
- Her timetable for when to take what medication left by her bed.
- The hall cleared of anything she might trip over on her way to the toilet.

On and on the list goes. I sigh as I head through to the sitting room and allow my body to crumple for the first time today. I keep the volume on the TV low in case Joyce needs me. I lean my head back on the couch and stare up at the ceiling, so that I don't have to look at the pile of mail on the table that contains all the bills for Joyce's treatment. I close my eyes, feeling utterly jaded. I can't stand to think any further.

I wake with a jerk, my hand springing to my neck as pain shoots upwards from my sudden movement. I glance to the door half expecting to see Joyce clinging to it, needing help for something but she's not there … she never is anymore. I put the TV on mute just in case and then I hear a small bang … bang … bang. I leap up and head straight to Joyce's room but it's empty. Without thinking, I go to the bathroom – that's the only other place she'll realistically be.

'Joyce, are you ok?' I call through the door.

There's no reply, only another bang.

'I'm coming in ok,' I warn, fingers tensed around the door handle.

I push open the door with numb hands, afraid of what I'll find.

'Joyce,' I whisper, the words snatched away from me as I take in the sight of her crumpled body sat on the toilet seat.

I step into the bathroom, my eyes taking in the liquid at her feet as she sits on the toilet having reached it too late. Her body doubled over, the weight of it supported by the bath which runs along the side the toilet – a small bottle of soap in her hand as she gives one last feeble bang with it.

'Joyce,' I say breathlessly, crouching down beside her.

She lifts her head a little, her unwashed hair falling across her face in clumps.

'I … I couldn't,' she tries but the effort drains her further.

'It's ok.'

'… in time,' she says, her voice so small and childlike.

'It's ok,' I say again. I wrap my arms around her hunched form and together we weep, neither of us wanting to see the other cry.

'Come on, let's get you cleaned up,' I say, looking around the bathroom and wondering just how I'm going to achieve this. 'Are you ok here?'

I take her silence as confirmation. I head to the utility room and grab the metal stool before carrying it back to the bathroom.

'Ok, if you sit on this then we can get you cleaned up,' I tell her gently.

I help her to move from the toilet to the stool which I've placed by the sink. Her body still doubled over as though she's permanently bent in the middle.

'Do you want to sit up?' I ask.

She doesn't say anything but she does try to straighten up a little. I put one arm across her chest and the other on her lower back – cautiously pushing and pulling my arms together. I hesitantly release the pressure once she's straighter and leaning up against the wall of the bathroom. Her face is shockingly pale, her lips and hands tainted blue. I can even see the blue of the veins across her face. I wonder how much she can see. Her eyes are so swollen and bruised looking, it's as though she's been beaten by the ghost of exhaustion. I watch the rise and fall of her collarbones as she struggles to catch her breath and as I realise my mistake.

'I'm sorry, Joyce, you're going to have to stand up. I should have taken your pyjamas down before you sat. I'm sorry,' I say, 'I'm so sorry.'

I take her under one of my arms and gently heave her

upwards. I can feel her muscles trembling within my arms as I quickly pull down her trousers and let her collapse the few inches she was able to stand. I dump the dirty garments in the bath – hiding them from view. Filling the sink with warm soapy water, I soak a facecloth from the cupboard underneath it.

'No,' Joyce begs almost inaudible, as she tried to recoil from me but has no physical strength to do so.

'I have to,' I tell her desperately, pulling down her t-shirt to cover her decency.

She instantly seems less distressed but silent tears fall from her eyes. I try not to think how degrading this must be for her as I wipe the facecloth over her skin.

'Is your skin sore?' I ask, watching as tears spill over her eyes.

She nods almost imperceptibly. I try to be as gentle as I can but, although she never complains, I can tell the soft fabric still hurts her. I bite the inside of my mouth. Hating that I'm hurting her further. I give up, and instead I simply squeeze the water over her legs and feet, the water soaking into my slippers as it spreads out in an uneven pool around us. Joyce just sits there, her eyes glazed over. I've never seen someone look so shut down. To live with so little life. She no longer cries. She just stares with deadened eyes into the nothingness. I look at her blank face, more scared of the scars this disease is leaving on her mind than on her body. I listen to the trickle of the water as it falls from the cloth, glides over the curves of her skin-covered bones and drips onto the floor. The scant muscles she worked so hard to regain now gone.

'Ok,' I say quietly. 'That's your legs and feet clean. If I stand you up and I hand you the cloth, do you want to try to clean yourself?'

She simply sniffs.

'I …' she sighs, as though she can't take the weight of everything within her. The words that come after come out as a whisper. 'Don't want … you … to see.'

'I won't look, I promise,' I tell her.

It's a lie, I have to look, I have to watch her movements to make sure she's keeping her balance. To judge when she sways from fatigue; which way I need to hold her to counter the movement as she tries to clean herself. Once she's done, I sit her back on the chair and drape a towel around her legs and across the soaking floor before I get her clean clothes. I hate having to ask her to get back up again, so that I can pull her bottoms up but, once I get them on, we make the painfully slow process from the soggy bathroom floor to her room, her feet shuffling along the ground – her body so sick she can hardly lift them. I lift her legs into the sofa bed for her. Feeling my face tense as she tries to push herself backwards so that she can sit up in bed, the pain in her eyes like a wound to my own, I gently nod as she succeeds – an absurd sense of pride filling me for this pathetically momentous achievement.

'Do you need anything else?' I ask, as Dog slips through the door and gently climbs into bed alongside her.

'No,' I lip-read from her.

I nod before tentatively rearranging her pillow, desperate to feel like I'm doing something to help. I look at her tiny frame, so fragile and frail. I gently run my hand over her head, aware of the tangled strands which are coming away under my fingers, but that's not why I gently pull away. She doesn't say anything but I can tell by the tensing of her jaw that my gesture hurts her. I clasp my hands together, the tender instrument of her pain; stroking her hair was the only thing that comforted her as a child and now I can't even do that. I glance around the room once more before heading to the hall. I close the door, my hand clasped over my mouth so she can't hear my cry.

Chapter Seven

JOYCE – AGE 23

The medication timetable of the sick:
- An hour before breakfast
- Breakfast
- An hour after breakfast
- An hour before lunch
- Lunch
- An hour before tea
- Tea
- An hour after tea (no hot liquids allowed)
- An hour before bed
- Bed
- An hour after bed

Seconds turn into days and days pass into weeks – they're stubborn like that but I fail to notice their changing. We, the sick, don't calculate time – instead we calculate moments and how much surviving them will cost us. So instead, in the months after my treatment ends, I simply strive to relearn how to feed myself, how to bathe, how to walk. It's hard to comprehend that I'm an adult when I'm infantile ... truly I'm neither. You'd think after three rounds I'd have recovery down to a fine art, and in a way I do. I know what baby steps to take but I also know that each step will only lead me to another and another and how long and how hard I will have to fight to take each one.

Imagine something you've devoted your life to, sacrificed the things you adore for, absorbed your every thought and emotion and passion into. Something that you've pushed yourself so hard to achieve that you felt like it'll break you ... now imagine the thing you fear the most in this world smashing it to pieces. Of having to painstakingly rebuild that creation all over again – only for the same thing to happen again and again and again. Imagine that dream wasn't a dream at all but instead your life. Tell me, at what point would you stop?

'Have you been outside today?' Aunt Beth asks that evening, as we sit in front of the TV.

'No.' My voice comes out cracked; I can't remember the last time I used it.

'Have you tried going outside yet? Last time you came off treatment you were ...' she pauses, perhaps sensing the danger in her words. 'You've been off treatment for months now. Maybe you should try going outside. Maybe see if you can make it to the bench and then go a step further each day? I know it's hard but it's the only way to start progressing,' she suggests tentatively.

I ignore her, determinedly not looking at her even though I know she's watching me for a reaction. You don't have a clue, I say inwardly. You have a clearer idea than most, and yet you're ignorant.

'Joyce,' Aunt Beth says with a hint of frustration, turning the volume on the TV down – which for her must make it mute although I can still hear the voices of the actors.

I try to pull myself off the couch but my excuse of a body fails me. Trembling, panting, pain shooting up my legs, I fall back onto the couch. I'm like a lump of cement attempting to be held up by sticks. Aunt Beth no longer hastens to help me, she takes her time getting up; the shock value has worn off after so many years of living like this. With an arm around my waist and another under my arm, she helps me to my feet and to walk the short distance from the sitting room to my dining room. I hate this cottage. I hate its stone walls, built brick by brick to cage me and yet I daren't try to escape it.

Dog comes bounding after us; launching himself onto my sofa bed before I can reach it and settling himself on the side of the bed designated as his. Aunt Beth deposits me and pulls up the covers.

'Thank you,' I say gratefully, but the words feel and taste as bitter as clotted blood.

I resent her; I need her. I loathe the reason why.

She nods, clearly not knowing what else to say.

'Need anything?' she adds, looking around the room for ungiven clues.

'No.'

Aunt Beth shuts the door and leaves me and Dog alone. He lifts his head and drops it onto my lap, the only weight pressed upon me that ever feels like comfort, his big brown eyes gazing up at me until I have no choice but to relent to the feeble smile hidden within me.

I look at the closest of the two bookcases which line either side of the fireplace, my eyes lingering on a piece of coral Logan found at the beach. It was after my first round of treatment and he spent ages talking me into leaving the house. We had the entire beach to ourselves. It was like the world was ours and ours alone.

I sat on the golden sand, the weight of my body sinking into it, like a seat made just for me. The glowing sun flitted between clouds of the purest white as Logan and Dog ran after each other like children playing tig. I close my eyes in my dark and dingily lit dining room, trying to replay the movements of my two best friends as they ran across the beach, trying to remember the sensation of the warmth of the sand as I held it in my palm and slowly let it sink through my fingers or simply the sound of the waves. Those beautiful white horses charging up the beach to tickle my toes. I try to remember the feeling I felt of knowing that something good was happening, the feeling of confirmation that this was why I had endured so much but all I can remember now is the months leading up to it and now all the months I have to relive once more.

How many months did it take to regain the strength to wash myself; first with a facecloth and with my aunt washing my hair over the sink and then in the shower? We've learned from past mistakes after the time I couldn't get up off the shower tray where I sat to wash … I now have a stool. I can't remember now how long it took to go from washing one dish at the sink a day until I could wash the lot. I still remember the first time I was well enough to make myself something to eat … the taste of it didn't live up to the effort it took to make. I know it was more than three months before I was able to walk out the back door. Painstakingly, each and every day, walking just one pathetic step more until I could reach the bench. The thought of pushing my body to do the things it feels incapable of doing, until it's capable once more, of brutally forcing myself through the pain when my body is screaming out to rest … is more than I can take.

'I'll start again tomorrow,' I say to Dog.

He looks at me … we both know it's a lie.

I sit in the window seat of my bedroom upstairs, still trying to regain my breath from the dizzying hike up here. Dog's head resting on my lap as I gaze out at the mountains, the first covering of early snow like a velvet hat on their peaks. I turn my head away from them … I can hardly remember what it feels like to walk up them now.

I keep coming up here, now that I can manage the stairs, in the hope that if I spend time in this room it'll start to feel more like mine but it never does. I am an intruder. A passing and unwanted guest. I don't even have the outward body of the girl I used to be. My skin's no longer so taut, unblighted; I have fractures from where I frown. I evade all mirrors, if I can, because I don't recognise who I've become. I've aged nearly seven years in what may as well be seven days.

I know it annoys Aunt Beth that I haven't moved up here. She keeps asking when I go to bed if I'd like to try the stairs. Aunt Beth doesn't dare say it but I know she thinks I've given up. She's wrong of course, I can't give up because I had nothing left to give up on in the first place. After all this time and after everything that's happened … I'm afraid that I've forgotten what it is to live.

I watch my hand as I stroke Dog's head. Aunt Beth has been so busy recently that he's not been getting out nearly as much as he should. He's generous with us, he's far better behaved than we deserve for him to be. I can feel his boredom though, how his eyes watch Aunt Beth with faltering hope as she comes home from work and sinks onto the couch with exhaustion – he gave up looking to me for excursion a long time ago.

'I'm sorry,' I whisper. This isn't the life any of us wanted.

I curl one knee up to my chest and wrap my arm around it, forcing myself to stay for just a moment longer. The weight of the life that once lived in this room is so vast that it consumes mine a thousand times over. I can't bear to remember the person I've lost and yet I'm terrified of forgetting because once I do … what will I have left? When a life so big now contains so little, your only choice is to depend on memories in order to remind you of what you're fighting for in the first place. But memories are cruel. They fade. And, with their departure departs the foundations on which you were counting on to rebuild your life. Memories become a mirage, then a myth and a legend until it seems impossible that those memories could belong to you. Because how on earth could that person have ever been so happy?

Chapter Eight

BETH

The top hacks to living with the chronically sick.

1. Embrace – any aid which can make your life easier, be it technological or emotional.

2. Relish – your guilty pleasures. These are your little breaks, your escape! Even if it's a programme you'd never admit to watching in public, a nap or downing a whole bottle of wine ... well, the latter should really just be wishful thinking but sometimes needs must.

3. Eat well – living on convenience, caffeine, sugar boosts and booze will only get you so far. You need to look after yourself, otherwise how can you look after those who are sick?

4. Exercise – same logic as above ... besides, I think we all know the importance of it.

5. Organisation – save yourself from panicking and fretting. Retaining all medical information about said sick person, in one, two, three, four ... ok, sometimes up to five fat folders saves a lot of stress and mess later on. Plan at least two days in advance so that you can cook ahead, buy booze ahead (again wishful thinking ... we all have our fantasies) and order medication etc.

6. Ask for help – presuming you actually have any, take it on behalf of all of us who don't and by all means don't ever abuse it.

7. Let yourself feel – you're allowed to grieve; you're allowed to be sad and you're allowed to show it. You've lost something, too.

8. The burnout – have you ever seen a hamster run so fast on its wheel that it catapults itself off it? The burnout is a little like that; you're frantically racing to do everything but, at some point, you come flying off and stun yourself into not being able to do anything at all. So, follow the hacks above to help prevent it!

9. Support groups – I hear are supportive. I personally find them depressing … but why not give it a go.

10 Remember – to actually act upon your hacks.

I pull into the drive and turn off the engine – the sudden silence somehow less peaceful than the noise. A lone leaf falls into my windshield, listless and shrivelled up by winter's approach. I sit for a while, enjoying the simple sensation of knowing that I can turn on the engine and leave. I think of all the places I could go; I don't particularly care where so long as it's far from here, somewhere where no one needs me, somewhere I can think solely of myself and do whatever I want … I sigh heavily, I can never decide if a fantasy is a mercy or a master criminal of hope.

Reluctantly, I grab my jacket from the passenger seat and head inside. Kicking off my boots in the darkened utility room at the back door, not bothering to turn on the light, I pause on the threshold into the kitchen. Its surfaces are illuminated by the dull lights under the cabinets above them. My eyes search for any manifestation of change, for the slightest of alterations on how I left it this morning ... but there are none. I cross my arms in front of my chest and hold onto my shoulders as I sigh; the newfound weight in my chest hard to dispel. I wander to the sink and stare dejectedly at my dirty dishes from this morning. I keep leaving them here in the hope that Joyce will put them into the dishwasher while I'm at work.

It was the little things for me, which were the giant things for her, which created the building blocks of her recovery after every round of treatment. The movement of washing a dish, which to someone who only recently couldn't lift their arm to feed themselves, was a momentous task. It was an achievement to be proud of, even if she never saw it that way. I understand the degradation it inflicted upon her but still she washed that single dish each day – until, slowly, she washed them all. Everything progressed from there. Only, it isn't happening that way this time.

I pick up my cereal bowl and hold it in my hand, the cold ceramic clutched within my fingers, staring at, yet utterly without seeing, the left-over cereal sludge at the bottom – congealed milk with flecks of cereal floating like drowned bodies in a sea of white blood.

She's making progress, I have to remind myself, but it's slower than it has ever been before. I feel like her improvements stem from the natural growth of coming off treatment; rather than a result of her intervention and encouragement. I open the dishwasher and, glad that I forked out to replace the broken one, I shove my dishes inside it, shutting the door with unnecessary force so that the tray of glasses shudder in a clinking cacophony. It's odd how we take out our pain on the things which support us the most.

I catch sight of my reflection in the kitchen window before me. The sight of my ageing body never fails to surprise me. It's like the last seven years have gone and I never paused to notice their passing … if only the deepening lines on my face had taken the same stance as I did. I take my hair out of the messy bun I hastily shoved it into earlier, remembering how luxurious it used to feel, as my fingers get caught in knots and as plaster dust coats my fingers. I give up and scrape it back into a bun.

I tear my eyes away from my reflection and try to focus on the kitchen around me and the things which need doing. Because, somehow, we always carry on. The motions are gone through. The requirements of the day are met or at least attempted. I take our dinner out of the slow cooker which, along with the dishwasher, has become my greatest ally. I prepare our food the night before and put a reminder on my phone to remind Joyce to turn it on the next day, followed by a second reminder an hour later – in case she forgets. Occasionally, I pretend that all the kids are home and they've made this surprise meal for me, like they sometimes did when they were young and cooking was a novelty rather than a nightly chore, all of them working in unison for a single act of kindness just for me.

'Hi,' I say, catching sight of Joyce by the door into the kitchen.

'Dog needs walked, he's been pacing all day,' Joyce informs me.

I'm fine thanks Joyce, how are you? Yes, my day was very stressful but at least it was productive; how was your day? Plays the conversation in my head.

'Your dinner's ready,' I remark despondently, turning back round to the slow cooker.

'Thanks,' she mutters, coming over and taking the fine bone china plate I hand her.

The china plate's lighter than the rest and this small alteration in weight can make the difference between her being strong enough to carry it herself … another small trick to aid the illusion of independence.

We eat in the sitting room while watching TV, allowing the noise of the fictitious and superior lives of others to fill the room.

'Sarah was asking after you,' I try an hour later once dinner is done but Joyce simply nods. 'She said she'd not heard from you in a while.'

'Can I get a shower?' she asks, ignoring my comment.

'Yes,' my answer comes out as a sigh. 'Do you need a hand?'

Joyce shakes her head. She's like a child who lost her favourite toy; shrunken, dejected and aimless. She manages to get up from the couch unaided and shuffles out the room like an elderly hunchback – too weak to hold herself fully upright. I look away. It physically pains me to watch her.

'Remember to leave the door unlocked,' I call after her.

I listen to the bathroom door shut and a moment later the splatter of the water hitting the tray before it settles into a steady flow. I stare at the picture on the mantlepiece, of the four of us all squished together, with me on the left followed by my daughter Kate, then Joyce's little sister Sarah and Joyce herself at the end. None of us are looking at the camera; instead we're looking at each other, our faces bunched with laughter in a rare moment where we all found joy. Sarah gave me that picture last year for Mother's Day – to me, it will always be the last trip we took before our lives changed irrevocably. My eyes linger on Joyce's bright face. I keep losing her. With each round of treatment, the girl that starts to form substance reverts back into shadow and I with her.

I used to get annoyed at Joyce for pushing herself so hard after her treatment ended. She was so determined to get better that she often made herself ill in the process of recovering ... I never understood that the opposite could be so much worse. Perhaps she's come to the conclusion that there's no point in trying or maybe she's afraid that, once she starts improving and finally gets to the stage where she's making real progress, they'll put her back on treatment like they have every time before.

I involuntarily shudder ... each of those options has a damming conclusion for us both. I don't blame her. After all, how many times can a child voluntarily be forced to plunge themselves back into the depth of their deepest dread? How many years and how many tears can fall for that slightest shimmer of hope to appear, only for it to be snatched away? How much can one person take before they break?

It's an effort to take my eyes off the picture, to return to reality because reality's not a place I want to be anymore. My eyes don't want to be forced away from a memory of a moment in which we were all so happy ... but forced away they are.

I get up and head into the hall, pausing to knock on the bathroom door.

'Joyce, how are you managing ... Joyce?'

I knock on the door again, only with more force and urgency, my gut-clenching at thoughts of her having fallen.

'Joyce, if you don't answer me, I'm going to open the door!'

I listen as the flow of water slowly dies away as though someone has turned off the rain and a small voice, previously unheard over the torrent, tells me she's fine.

I drag my feet to the utility room to hang up the washing I put on last night. Flicking on the light, I halt at the sight before me. The airer is standing in the corner as normal but with two of its three tiers covered in clothes; the basket sitting next to it partly empty. I stare at it, my rational brain trying to repel my hope because I'm certain this partial act wasn't conducted by me. I kneel on the floor by the horrible, cheap, grey basket which now contains the evidence of a lavish attempt of effort. I sit there, staring at the airer for so long that the chill in the tiles is replaced by my body's warmth. I raise my hand to cover my mouth as though if anyone sees my growing smile then this will all disappear and this single moment, in now nearly seven months of despair, will have never been. I wipe my eyes, my heart swelling with pride as I take in each and every item hanging on the line.

Unthinkingly, I hasten to my feet at the sound of the bathroom door opening. I almost collide into Joyce as she enters the hall with a towel wrapped tightly around her bony frame. She hardly has time to see I'm there before I hug her and simply hold her against me, her arms at her side as though unsure of what to do with them. Her wet hair, warm from the shower, soaking into my top.

'You're incredible, you know that,' I tell her.

She doesn't say anything but I feel a small hand, like a child's, clutching the back of my top as though she's trying to keep her tired arm up in order to hug me back.

Chapter Nine

JOYCE – AGED 23

I glare at my aunt's breakfast dishes from across the kitchen table. I know she leaves them there on purpose. On that principle alone, I refuse to clear them away.

I return my attention to the jigsaw before me. I've learned, with reluctance, that these puzzles are not simply something with which to pass the time but a full-on, hardcore, upper body workout. The lifting of heavy arms to chest height, the extension to reach for the dumbbell of a carboard puzzle piece, the tremble-inducing hover over the square frame (because only the reckless start without putting the edges together), the flexibility and yoga for stiffened fingers as they shift the dumbbell about trying all four or, if it's a really wild piece, five sides before giving up and searching for another. At first, I could only manage three pieces at a time before my back sagged and the burning in my arms refused further strain ... I still resent the pain, which is yet to be worth the gain.

I pause to examine the picture, it was Aunt Beth who bought it – meant as a kind gift, a well-done for surviving another round of treatment ... I now have the full collection.

'You look as fed up as I feel,' I tell Dog, sitting back in my chair, which he's lying next to.

He sits up and slowly jumps up onto his hind legs, his two

front paws resting on the edge of my seat, his cold wet nose nuzzling under my tired arm until his hairy head is holding up my arm like he's my personal armrest.

'What?' I ask, my voice taking on an involuntary gushiness that I can't resist with him.

He headbutts my arm until it falls away, his tail swinging hypnotically round like a helicopter's propeller.

'Ok, down now,' I tell him, his eyes boring into mine as we have a stare down. 'Dog, down. Stop!'

I pull my arm back as his blunt but piercing claws scrape at my arm – leaving four red welts on my blue tainted skin. He looks at me utterly uncaring before pushing himself off my chair and moving to sit at the back door expectantly. I sigh as I push my chair back, feeling the internal reverberation of my spine and shoulders popping as I get to my feet to open the door for Dog to go into the garden.

He steps over the threshold and then sits on the top step; staring at me as though waiting for me to join him in the bitterly cold air.

'Go,' I order him, trying to shift his fluffy tail out of the way with my foot, but every time I shift it to safety it reflexes back over the threshold.

I give up and return to my seat at the table, the cold air from outside stalking my steps. I try to ignore him but I can feel him watching me.

'What?' I ask, as though he can answer.

In a way, his whine affirms what I already know.

'I can't,' I whisper, pleading for him to understand.

Dog launches himself through the utility, his claws scrabbling across the tiles in the kitchen as he attempts to regain control before colliding with my chair and making me judder. He spins around three, four times before racing back out the door.

He whines beggingly at me again and I feel my body sag, only this time it's not from fatigue but from failure. I stare at the world beyond him, his ears framing the view my eyes settle on.

You could take him out. You could try, a voice whispers in my mind. I stand up and move towards the back door carefully, curiously but mostly cautiously, as though someone might come up behind me and push me through the vortex of the back door. The sky is darkening, the scant sun of winter's afternoon already beginning to fade away. I look towards the gate at the end of the garden, captured within an arch of unkempt hedging, the field beyond it enticing yet looming with danger. It doesn't seem real somehow. It's as though I'll get to the gate and the view I've been staring at all these years will be nothing but a paper cut-out, with nothing behind it but deepening depths of darkness.

'I can't,' I tell Dog, feeling my eyes widen from within.

My eyes dart around the garden, certain that someone is hiding, waiting for me to come outside and … and do what I don't know, but I know I won't like it. I taste blood long before I feel the pain of biting the inside of my cheeks. I know I'm being stupid; I know it's irrational, I know it's not me but, like this disease, I can't get it out of me; we are one and the same, each created and cultivated to try and one up the other in dominance. We both fight and strive to live the best life we can. Strangely, it's this realisation which steadies me … the best life that I can have.

I glance back at the partially completed jigsaw; picturing myself sitting there five years from now. The very real reality that I could be that person for the rest of my life terrifies me.

I look into Dog's hopeful eyes.

'Ok,' I whisper meekly. 'We can do this ... we can do this, right?' I say to him, repeating the words as though they'll fortify me.

I shuffle around the cottage, putting on a hat, jacket and gloves. I pause before taking off my gloves to put on my boots, as and when I come across them, the normal order of dressing so long forgotten it needs thought. I take my walking stick from the umbrella stand by the front door – it's really a mountaineering pole but, like a lot of things I bought before I was ill, its use and name has been redefined.

By the time I'm ready to walk out the door, I'm already flagging from the exhaustion of getting ready. My body begs me to return to my sofa bed but, after all the effort it's taken to get ready, I refuse not to try.

I lower myself onto the back step, the cold air wrapping me in its icy arms, as Dog jumps up and down on his front paws as though he's clapping the ground to applaud me onwards. My hesitant feet crunch down onto frostbitten grass, those fragile fragmented crystals crushing and cementing into footprint after footprint, stick print after stick print ... evidence of my efforts.

Dog bounds alongside me as we approach the gate into the field, my thickly gloved fingers rushing to unbolt the gate before I have time to think about what I'm doing. I hold my breath nonetheless, certain that as soon as I step through the paper view that I'll fall into nothingness, but of course I don't. I step onto frostbitten grass, which is longer and coarser than that of the garden. I look around for Dog, my heart lurching when I find him missing. But he's sitting by the gate looking at me with his pink tongue peeking out from between his dark muzzle.

'Come, Dog,' I invite, clapping my free hand to my thigh,

forgetting that he needs permission to leave the garden – I feel like we both do.

My grip tightens on my stick as Dog eagerly rushes towards me and then past me. The darkness shielding me from the non-existent eyes I can feel watching me, judging me, waiting to assault or accost me. My fingers ache under the vice grip I hold onto my stick with. I'm hyperaware of everything around me, my body so stiff and rigid that even the sight of a bird taking flight makes my heart lunge. I watch my feet as I take my next tentative step away from the gate, my eyes studying the frozen grass as it's compressed beneath my feet, both so soft and solid at the same time.

As I make my way further from the house, Dog's legs leap liberally through the long tangle of sagging grass, while mine languish, stumble and stall. I watch as ghosts run rings around me. Memories of us as children cycling our bikes in this field fill my sight. I watch the space ahead of me as Sarah and Kate climb a tower of now non-existent hay bales, yelling for me to join them. My legs momentarily flourish in the memory. Their impulse to run almost makes me think that I can. I look down at my spindly legs as the instinct is overtaken by the aching in every one of my joints. When I look back up, I'm alone.

My eyes linger on the old fence post Sarah, Kate and I used to race to as kids and I make it my target. I pause, three posts away from it, my legs humming with the effort each step is costing me. I keep my eyes on the post ahead of me though, it's identifiable from the rest by it being thicker and rounder – more like a telegraph pole. As kids, the first to reach it and sit on its top was the winner, bruises were frequently incurred … we didn't always play fair. Dog comes racing up to me, his nose nuzzling against my hand.

'I'm ok,' I assure him, though warm tears turn to cold streaks upon my cheeks as I pat his head.

He looks up at me for a moment as though assessing the validity of my words before sprinting off again.

'I can do this,' I order resentfully, my body screaming at me to stop.

Slowly, my laboured legs take me closer to my target. My gloved hand reaching for it beseechingly, my wooden life vest, I'm desperate for it to save me. I wrap my outstretched arm around it as my chest collides into the wooden post, my legs barely there to hold me upright. My misted breath melting the ice covering the post as I try to catch the cold air in my lungs, my eyes blurring ... all I can think is that I made it. I actually made it.

'We did it,' I exclaim breathlessly to Dog, who's watching me from further up the field, but as I look around me my voice slowly fades into nothing because what should feel like a victory now doesn't ... it feels almost pathetic. I'm not even 200 yards from the gate.

I try to remember what the feeling of accomplishment is like, I try to make myself feel it but I don't know how and somehow that leaves me feeling emptier than before. I try to put a name to what I think I feel; as I realise that this is the first time I've left the house alone in at least seven years, but still, I feel ... nothing.

I look round me, the skeletons of once leafy trees now bare and bland, glowing white in the moonlight, which the encroaching darkness is making all the brighter.

I can't, I can't do this, I sink my head to my hand as though to shield myself from the shame I can't yet feel. This isn't me. Surely this isn't me. I'm desperate to sit down but I'm not foolish enough to believe that I can get back up. I'm shattered and broken in more ways than I thought it possible to be. My aloneness is more than my heart can take. My future bleaker than it was when I was dying because at least then I had something to fight for.

I want to let my legs give way, to collapse to the ground and stay there, for the sun to come up and melt me into the ground until there's nothing left. I cling to that choice until my legs start to feel less like the fragile flakes of ice all around me. I can barely see Dog as he comes racing up to me, he jumps onto his hind legs so that his front paws are resting on the post and pants onto my face.

I lean away from his grinning muzzle to bury my face in his neck as he rubs his head across mine.

Reluctantly, I unbury myself from Dog's comfort, grip my stick tightly in one hand and release myself from my life vest … wading back into the treacherous waters to try to get home, my anchor to this world keeping pace alongside me.

Two days later, it's Dog's unrelenting pestering which drags me out into the darkness once more. He started his campaign of unrelenting irritation at noon but I held out until it started to get dark – too afraid to leave without its concealment. There was a small flurry of snow which swayed in the wind as I clung to my post for longer than I needed to, just to watch the flakes dance before me, to feel them tickle my skin as they landed on the only parts of me not covered in thermals. Their frozen beauty melting into nothingness – it seems wasteful that something so beautiful could disappear in an instant.

The day after that, Dog seemed to expect me to take him out and my guilt at not doing so eventually dragged me back to my post and then beyond it. While I trudged through each painstaking step, I debated with myself over telling Aunt Beth but I know she won't like it. I can see the worry on her face though, thinking I'm regressing, because I'm so weak again in the evenings now ... she doesn't know it's a consequence of walking Dog. It's not fair, but how else am I meant to progress? Besides, I like the sense of secrecy, of having something no one else knows. I treasure my secret like a priceless jewel – relishing having something no one else can have. It's my one tiny piece of control.

In the following weeks, it became the sense of entrapment inside the tiny cottage, along with Dog's expectations, that pushes me from my cage. At the weekend, it starts to irk me that I can't go for my walk because Aunt Beth will find out. Come Monday, I'm waiting with almost as much anticipation as Dog is for the darkness to arrive.

Dog's eagerness, his sheer joy of being outside and of having me with him, is what makes me take that extra step when I think there's nothing left inside me to give ... until slowly, so terribly slowly, I begin to find the joy in it too. And in a bid to keep it, I'm reluctantly willing in the passing months and in the ever-lightening skies of spring ... to risk being seen by all.

Chapter Ten

BETH

I pause as I enter the function room of the hotel, the sea of bodies choppy and unstable as I try to pick out the person I'm here to see. The noise from each person rumbling over the other. The mission: say hi to Jimmy, give him his gift ... don't get caught.

'Beth!' says a loud and drawling female voice from behind me.

My shoulders deflate with defeat as I recognise the voice. I turn around to see the secretary from the company I used to work for standing behind me. Her perfectly bobbed hair is dyed an unnatural shade of blond, given how dark her eyebrows are. Steph, a kind lady with views higher than her station, had always been nice to me but her sharp eyes have always reminded me of a crow – forever peering and pressing to gain more information than you were ever comfortable to give.

'Steph, how are you?' I ask.

'Wonderful, I'm just back from holiday and I'm retiring soon too,' she gushes, running her hand up and down her bare arm to highlight her tan. 'And, how are you? Still working for yourself?'

I glance around the bustling room, wondering if I can drag someone else into the conversation, but everyone is occupied. My eyes catch sight of the long banner above the door of the hotel's function room, which reads, 'Jimmy, you might be retiring but you've not lost your spanners yet!'

'I'm good, thanks. Happily working for myself … my only problem is finding time for all the jobs I have on the go,' I throw in for good measure.

'Really,' she says, her neck extending towards me like a chicken on the hunt for grain. 'Must be hard, all that work while looking after a sickly child. How is Janice these days? Did they ever find out what was wrong with her?'

'You know, *Joyce* is making leaps and bounds,' I say, before I can stop myself. 'If you'll excuse me, I need to say hi to Jimmy.'

I swiftly turn and walk away as Steph opens her mouth to reply. As I walk past the drinks table, I grab a glass of apple juice … wishing it was wine.

I hang back for a moment, until Jimmy finishes his conversation, before going up to him.

'Beth, I'm so glad you could make it,' Jimmy says warmly, extending his arms for a hug.

'I wouldn't have missed it for the world,' I say, hugging him back before handing him a gift bag. 'Congratulations on retiring. I hope you like it.'

Jimmy sneaks a peek inside before looking up at me, his eyes alight.

'You didn't!' he says.

'It's not much,' I confess, suddenly aware of the large table overflowing with far larger gifts than mine.

'Are you kidding … I've been given enough booze to outdrink the navy and not one gift has been as thoughtful as this,' he says, pulling out the pair of slippers which have written on each their designated foot.

'Well, you complained enough about putting them on the wrong feet when we worked together,' I remind him, smiling at his reaction.

'Thank you!' he says, with a laugh. 'Still can't believe I'm retiring.'

'Me neither,' I say. He's younger than me, after all. 'Enjoy the rest of your party.'

'Keep in touch,' he calls as a small group of people start vying for his attention.

I intended to go straight home but I couldn't quite bring myself to. Instead, I park at the nearby loch and sit. I blink, my eyes unseeing. The compact dirt path beneath my feet hardly seems to be there at all. My knees ache from the weight of my elbows, which rest upon them, as I lean forward like a drunkard preparing to be sick but of course I'm not. I just wanted the world to not be so big for a moment. Taking a steadying breath, I sit up, my face feeling flushed from the rush of blood. I look at the loch, where the water sits so calm and still. Its peaceful tranquillity teases me with what I should feel but instead its calming effects simply bounce off my shield of festering failures.

I wish I hadn't gone to that wretched party. So many of my friends are planning retirement, their voices quick and eager, high in pitch from the excitement of what this new life will bring them. Retirement's not something I can even consider. My life savings are gone. My home re-mortgaged down to the last blade of grass. My credit cards at their limits. Everything spent on a child who is alive but can barely live.

I lift my head to the sky and close my eyes for a moment, wrapping my jacket more tightly around me against the cool breath of early spring, thinking of Kate. I hate to admit it but I envy my own child. I glance at the dark screen of my mobile, which Kate just called me on to tell me of her new job and of living in engaged bliss. The intrusive device sits on the bench beside me. It gives as much as it takes, and I can't take much more.

I shake my head … I don't know if I'm scolding myself or the world. Why do those who should be granted mercy not receive it?

I stand up so abruptly that I scare a nearby bird into the air, my movement cutting off my thoughts. I'm abruptly aware of the sweet scent of nearby flowers promising anew but only for those who can emerge having survived the storms of winter.

I wander around the edge of the water. I don't want to think, I don't want to feel, I just want stillness … just for a moment, just until I can catch my breath. I can't stop my mind from picking at my life, from dissecting it piece by miserable piece.

I know Joyce feels bad for it but, still, I'm the one bruised by her unpredictable moods. Sobbing like a child, desperately buried so deep in despairing depression that I'm scared I can't pull her out; before turning to snapping anger. The whip of her words cut me clean, even though they say nothing to hurt me. I prance around her, my mind aching from the exhaustion of trying to pick my way through the detonators of her moods. Although a part of me revels in it, in her having energy enough to be angry is a sign to rejoice at and yet it stings to be the one who's subject to it. I have to keep reminding myself to separate her from it, to keep reminding myself to hate the disease and not her. To tell myself that it's just like when they were kids and you could love the child but hate the behaviour.

Half an hour later, having reluctantly returned home, I move about the kitchen preparing myself a cup of tea.

'I'm home,' I say loudly, finally giving up on the urge to hold off letting Joyce know I'm back. 'Do you want a cup of anything?'

I wait, listening to the silence which makes this tiny cottage feel huge.

'Joyce?' I snap a little. Sometimes I can't help it, either.

I slam the cupboard door shut and stride down the hall to her dining room door before gently knocking on her door. When I hear no sound, I quietly open the door to find the covers pulled back and the bed empty.

'Dog?' I call with suspicion before calling him again, only this time a little louder. 'Dog.'

'You've got to be kidding me,' I hiss as the thought hits me. I race up the stairs. 'JOYCE!'

I go into every room but she's not in any of them. I head to Sarah's old room, which looks out over the garden, even though I'm sure I would have seen her when I drove in.

My body sways with the blood pulsating throughout my body, memories flashing through my mind of the last time she disappeared, one hand on my temple as I look frantically around me.

'JOYCE!'

I rage internally as I storm through to my room and look out the window in the hope of spotting her. The last time she disappeared Logan found her unconscious in a ditch.

I study the road to the left, which Joyce took the last time she vanished, but I can't see any sign of movement. I glare at the road, which weaves round to the right, as though I can somehow intimidate it into revealing her to me but of course it doesn't.

I'm trying to think through what to do next when, through the blossoming trees, a splash of red catches my eye. It disappears and reappears from behind a tree with the unmistakable companion of Dog in tow beside it.

I watch Joyce amble slowly along the road, her weight leaning heavily upon her stick, her figure getting clearer and more detailed the closer she gets. My fingers clutch onto the ledge of the windowsill like it'll somehow hold the image still before me.

My hands lurch forward as she stumbles. My fingers and knuckles crunching sickeningly as they knock off the glass as I try, impossibly, to catch her but she steadies herself … pauses and after a while she carries on regardless. I feel like a mother proudly watching their toddler take its first steps, my arms outstretched, waiting for the fall, only to discover that my arms are now empty and unneeded. Instead, I wrap my arms around the loss that's inside me. My anger so swiftly changing from awe to grief that it dazes me. I watch her as she gets closer to the boundaries of the cottage, aware of a churlish desire to hide up here, to not go down and praise her achievement.

I wait until she gets closer to the drive before heading downstairs. My body moving around the kitchen, my fingers numb to the items they touch. I brew us both a cup of tea and then take them outside. I sit on the bench, the warmth of the mugs almost painful in my cupped hands, awaiting her return. I've already drunk a good amount of mine by the time she appears round the side of the house.

Joyce stops so abruptly upon seeing me that she has to use her free arm to counter her balance. Her face is flushed from exertion, the colour in her cheeks almost as deep a red as the flecks in her hair. Her eyes won't meet mine. She looks caught, guilty but also defiant. Slowly, she bends over to unclip Dog from his lead and he instantly comes bounding over to me. I clap him for a moment before looking up to see Joyce staring at me, twisting and untwisting the lead subconsciously in her hand. I watch her and she watches me while I internally fight the unexpected bitterness which wants to scold her. With a reluctant hand, I pat the space beside me on the bench and, hesitantly, she comes to the bench and sits beside me. I hand her a cup and we sit in mutual silence – neither of us having anything left to say to the other.

Chapter Eleven

JOYCE – AGE 23

The brutal rules of the recovering sick:

- Conserve energy – we ration everything. We have no choice. We don't walk, talk or do anything unless there's a point to it … the sick are more energy efficient than your lightbulbs.
- Selfishness – there are plenty of healthy humans who can lend a hand so you don't need to. I know, I know, we're terrible people but listen up, that five-minute favour can turn into an hour and that hour can turn into four days of recovery.
- Lists – write everything down because, let's face it, you're not going to remember otherwise. I'm not talking about a diary here (see rule 1), I'm talking bullet points in a notebook.
- Dedication – yeah, yeah, I know, you just want a day off, but suck it up, buttercup, because this disease isn't taking a break. You want to beat it, you need to give as good as you get in recovery. You need to push through the exhaustion, the pain, the tears … until the day comes when that small act which costs so much will suddenly cost less.
- Remember – to remember. This is also where your list comes in handy for proof. It's easy to forget, so take a moment … take it right now and remember how far you've come.

Don't let what those around you and what they're doing dampen your dreams. You're still here and that fact alone is incredible.

- Breathe – I know this will contradict point 4 but hear me out. We all know once you get a taste for life you don't want to stop, you want to reach the next rung in the ladder of recovery. It becomes compulsive, addictive, but you also can't afford to push yourself so hard that you break. So, know when to stop. To breathe. To pause. It's ok to take a day … a week and simply do nothing.
- Diet – yeah, yeah what's the harm in a bit of cake or fizzy juice … the answer … a lot! Tough it up – you're sick, you don't have the luxury of abusing your body if you want to get better. Our lives are not about choice and you can either punish your body for something that's not its fault or you can help it to heal by cutting out the crap.
- Stubbornness – is your greatest friend. Embrace it.

I still can't decide if Aunt Beth is proud or angry at me for secretly leaving the house each day. I think she's a mix of the two. I suspect she feels she can't tell me off because she's getting what she wanted, just not in the way she wanted it. Besides, I've found a new secret to hide from her. I became bored of walking. It's too slow, too mundane, so I've branched out into harder challenges. It came about as a result of the tragic demise of our old brick TV. I recoiled at first when Aunt Beth got the new one which connects to the internet. Somehow, it felt like an intruder to our sitting room, knowing that the companies who make them are gathering information and monitoring every click we make. Maybe it was my paranoia, but either way I didn't like it. Now I use the tv to execute my new daily dose of self-persecution.

I exhale through gritted teeth but refuse to surrender to the screaming in my thighs as I hold my squat, my eyes transfixed as my legs visibly tremble, like an earthquake building within me, until the structure breaks. I crumble, glutes first, to the sitting-room floor, pain shooting through my knees, my hip joints as gritty-feeling as gravel, my muscles so taut they feel like they might rip. I lie there, my heart lurching and pounding so hard that I'm scared it'll stop. Tiny fairy lights shimmer before my eyes as my sideways view of the room goes in and out of focus. The woman on the TV releases her squat hold and dives straight in for another.

'I know it's hurting,' she sighs over my music.

No kidding, I think bitterly.

'But this is our last one before we move on. Remember: only push yourself as far as you can go. It's important to push through but it's also important to know when to stop.'

I don't know when to stop, though, that's part of the problem and part of the result. It's the reason why I'm making such substantial improvements. As the woman on the TV lies on her mat and starts doing clamshells, I take a breath. Determined to sit up, determined that, one day, I'll complete this ten-minute video. I try to lift my head, which feels like a balloon of cement, off the floor, but I can barely lift it an inch. I try to sit up again but my arms tremble like a cowering pet before its abuser. I let my arms give in and I crumple back onto the floor. Slowly I curl myself into a ball, tears falling silently down my face. The consequences are more than I can bear. Yet still I do this every day. I push myself through the pain until I'm at the point of breaking. I pause only when my heart feels like it might cease to beat and my limbs give out from under me … otherwise, I don't stop, I can't.

I lie there, unmoving, ashamed of myself, of my weakness, of how hard everything in my life is, but mostly I'm scared that my life will forever be this.

The carpet prickles my skin as I try to remember what it used to feel like to work out; to run or cycle for miles on end. To feel my muscles humming from exhilaration. It was so easy, so fun, the aches and pains the next day were like impermanent victory scars but these scars, on an already shredded body, hold no sense of achievement.

I'm not sure if I fell asleep, or maybe I passed out. Either way, scraping myself up off the floor felt a lot like trying to peel superglue off my skin … resistant, reluctant and ultimately painful. I rest for a few hours before sitting at the kitchen table before another jigsaw. These mind-numbing games, I've learned, are not so mind-numbing after all and have become a part of my daily routine. I decided it's not enough to work out physically; this disease isn't just in my organs, muscle and bones after all. So, I use jigsaws to mentally work out, too – now I'm well enough to do more than place a couple of pieces at a time.

Apparently, jigsaws require the use of both sides of your brain. They enhance visual perception, coordination, improve memory, critical thinking and dopamine … although I find the last one questionable. It's safe to say I'm lacking in all these departments, thanks to my Lyme disease having a feast on my mental faculties: given the amount of dishware I chip and the bruises on my arms from walking into doors, I basically have no short-term memory or the ability to think in a functional manner, never mind a critical one and, let's not beat about the bush, I don't exactly have many feel-good feelings going on. So I'll reluctantly confess that these jigsaws are stimulating the growth of my cognitive function, now the treatment has reduced the Lyme's ability to tap dance on my brain cells.

My days, which so easily merge into one, consists of the same routine. I rely on it, depend on it and any disturbance within it can be disastrous to my ability to cope. Weekends are my enemy now because Aunt Beth is at home and there's no routine, no structure, no knowing what will happen at any given time.

And what do I get in return for this self-dictatorship? Well, I get to function around the house. Its maintenance is now back in my domain. And, occasionally, I get to re-emerge into the world. A world which is so foreign to me now that it may as well be a different country. A world so vast and fast that it terrifies me, but I'm getting better at it. I'm finding that as my body gets stronger, so does my courage for re-entering it.

Aunt Beth and I started off small. She started taking me for a drive each week to see how I would cope ... the answer, not well. I should have expected the results, given how hard I found it after my last treatments. Turns out that when your live your life at less than 3 mph, going into a metal contraption which travels at 70 mph has some rather unpleasant side effects. But, we worked on it and those drives grew longer and longer and then turned into trips to small coffee shops, those coffee shops turned into small shops and today I've been taken to what can only be described as the most mindbogglingly, overwhelmingly, gloriously gluttonous monstrosity I've been in in over seven years.

The shop's not busy but it's still too crowded for my liking. The place is crammed with products, literally, to the roof. As we wonder around the bargain store, Aunt Beth picks up this and that and drops the items into a trolley which is so deep we can barely touch the bottom. I trail after her like a toddler, my eyes moving this way and that – trying to take it all in. At home, I have the option of whatever Aunt Beth can get me – whether I like it or not. Most of the products I used before I was ill are either no longer in production or have changed so much in size, shape and description that they're no longer recognisable. It's been so long since I was well enough to be in a shop that I don't even know what the options are anymore. My eyes skim over five shelves dedicated solely to biscuits, the various colours and packaging pulling at my eyes, vying for my attention.

I lag behind Aunt Beth, who keeps watching me nervously, constantly assessing me to see how I'm coping, waiting for my body to start betraying warning signs that I'm not. She doesn't like that I now refuse to walk with my stick but we have an unspoken compromise in which she grumpily stashes it in the boot of the car when she thinks I'm not looking and I pretend not to notice.

We head into an aisle full of shampoo, bodywash and the like. I slowly turn around on the spot, submerged in a world of plastic, chemicals and artificial nonsense. It seems so unnatural that it's hideous. Did I never notice it before or was it so commonplace that I never questioned it?

'Do you think Sarah will like this?' Aunt Beth asks, holding up a bottle of lavender scented soap.

I shrug.

'Don't know …. Why are you getting her soap?'

'She's coming up to stay, remember?'

'Oh, yeah,' I mutter, watching as she drops the soap into the trolly, wondering why people always ask if you remember something you've obviously forgotten.

'What was it you needed?' Aunt Beth asks.

'I-ehh, I don't remember,' I tell her, trying to focus on her words and not the enormity of the things around me.

'I thought you wrote it down?' Aunt Beth reminds me.

'I did but I forgot the list,' I explain.

'Joyce,' Aunt Beth sounds, her shoulders sagging with frustration.

'I need toothpaste though,' I tell her, surprised by my own ability to recall that from the barren desert which is my mind.

'It's down there,' she tells me, pointing towards the end of the aisle.

I stare at the rows upon rows of toothpaste which whiten, brighten, remove stains, remove sensitivity, harden enamel and which taste minty, original, extra fresh ... on and on their credentials go. They all have such varying prices as well and all of them are far more expensive than I remember them being. I find I've no idea what a reasonable price for toothpaste is anymore. My eyes frantically move from one box to the next while I try to discern what I need or what kind I want but the number of options is baffling ... Why do we need so much choice? I pick up a box, stare at it, put it back, pick up another and then panic and go back to my original choice. I feel my body getting tighter and tighter as my muscles contract. I feel as though someone has a gun to two people and is asking me to pick which should live. It's just toothpaste, I remind myself, the world won't end if I pick the wrong one, and yet it feels like it will. I stare desperately between my various options; feeling like I can't breathe for the tightness in my chest.

'Is that the one you want?' Aunt Beth asks, holding out her hand to put it in the trolley.

'I don't know what to do,' I say beseechingly, my eyes stinging.

'About what?' Aunt Beth asks, stepping closer to me, her brow furrowed.

'I don't know what toothpaste to get.'

'Joyce,' she laughs, clearly expecting something more profound. 'It's just toothpaste, get the one you like.'

'It's not funny!' I nearly cry at her.

How can she think this is funny? I feel like my world will collapse with the incorrect answer. I can't do this. It's too much. It's too many things, too many people, too many options, too many prices, too many colours, it's just too many.

'Ok, I'm sorry,' Aunt Beth flusters to calm me. 'Why don't I help you?'

I nod submissively and she takes the toothpaste from my tighten grasp and examines it.

'Let's see what you've got,' she says placatingly. 'Well … this is denture cream so why don't we put it back.'

'It is?' I say in dismay.

'You'll glue your teeth together with this,' she says, hazarding a weary laugh.

I laugh half-heartedly, even though I don't feel like doing so, suddenly aware of how irrational my reactions are. Aunt Beth's presence has somehow shrunken the situation back down to its appropriate size and in turn I feel myself shrinking in shame.

Aunt Beth picks up two toothpastes and holds them out for me – I look at her blankly.

'Pick one,' she instructs.

'They both do the same things,' I tell her as I study them both. 'But, that one's a lot more expensive.'

'Ok, so we're going with the cheaper one?'

'But, what if the expensive one's better for my teeth?' I ask.

'Why don't you get both and then you'll know for future which one to get,' she says, with a hint of impatience.

I stare at her askance, my body automatically recoiling from the large man trying to get past us.

'I can't do that,' I say, although I've no idea why. 'I'll take this one … actually no, I'll take that one.'

'Ok,' Aunt Beth says.

'Wait,' I say, my panic rising once more – reaching out for my original pick. 'I want that one.'

As we head to the till, I glance judgmentally at the toothpaste sat amongst a jumble of other things … still unconvinced by my decision. By the time we reach the till, my back's aching and sagging, my knees biting with pain.

'If you had taken your stick, someone might have let us ahead of them,' Aunt Beth remarks, as she sees me holding onto the queue partition to steady myself.

She offers to take me to the car and then come back inside to pay for everything but I refuse her the satisfaction of being right. Besides, I've come this far, I want to see this through. As we reach the till and my items are scanned, I fluster for the money in my purse. For almost a decade now, whenever we've gone out, I've been ordered to sit while whoever I'm with makes the order. Logan always refuses to let me pay and I transfer whatever money I owe to Aunt Beth through my online banking. In the last seven years, I've had no dealings with physical money. I never thought it was a skill you could lose but, as the man on the till reads out how much I owe, I suddenly realise that all the notes and coins in my hand are meaningless. My heart thumps as I strain to remember if there's 60 seconds in a minute or if its 60p in a pound. I can feel the line of people behind me fidgeting impatiently as I stand there gormlessly. I hastily hand the man on the till all the notes in my purse. He looks at me oddly as he hands me back change, from the £40 I gave him, for my £7.83 purchases.

Once we get home, I examine the toothpaste I bought and decide, with a heavy heart, that I should have gone for the other one.

Chapter Twelve

JOYCE – AGE 23

It's been three days since I left the house ... three days! And not because I'm incapacitated, not because I don't want to, not because I can't but because of her. I know, two days to someone who has been housebound for close to a decade doesn't sound like much but I didn't have a choice back then, I physically couldn't leave, whereas this is enforced entrapment.

Sarah leans over to set a plate of food in front of me and then straightens up, waiting for my reaction. I look at the side serving of crisps next to the cheese and ham sandwich (which is made with my gluten-free bread and which has as much resemblance to bread as a deer does to a hamster but is better than nothing). She's cut the sandwich into four crumbly pieces like I'm a four-year-old who's a choking hazard.

'Thanks,' I mutter, looking up at her expectant face.

She's beautifully tanned, having just come back from being on holiday with all of her mates. The red pigments in her auburn hair, brighter after being in the sun, now rival my dull ones.

She returns to the counter to collect her plate. Her lunch also contains a sandwich which, I note, is only cut into two pieces.

Sarah sits down and we begin to eat but, after half a sandwich is consumed in silence, she picks up her phone which is sitting between us.

'Here, Jo sent me her holiday pictures this morning,' she says, holding the screen between us so that we can both see the image of her and her friends sitting, bleary eyed, in the airport holding up their coffee cups with the caption of: 'In need of the strong stuff … 4am start to our holiday.'

I momentarily close my eyes to block her out because the only thing more boring than seeing someone else's holiday pictures, when the new excitement of your life is being able to shower without being bedbound after … is seeing them for the third time only from a slightly different angle. And, of course, their presence requires the retelling of all the same stories I heard yesterday and the day before.

I was well behaved the first time. I gushed, I ooowed and awwwed, I gasped, I asked questions, I was the model sick sister. There was no chink in my armour of performance of faked interest and I won't deny I grew slightly curious at times. I'm glad she had a good time – at least, I'd never wish for anything else. But this is becoming cruel.

'And then Jo distracted the guy …'

'And you put Abby's number in his pocket,' I finish off, taking a bite from my disintegrating sandwich.

'Yeah,' she says, her elation at telling the story deflating at my words.

'So, did he message?' I ask, attempting to compensate for having just ruined her fun.

I sigh silently. I already know the answer.

'Of course he did!' Sarah gushes.

… but he turned out to be a weirdo, I finish the sentence off inside my head.

'But he turned out to be a total weirdo,' Sarah says, finishing off the last of the crisps on her plate.

See, my memory *is* improving, I reaffirm to myself – only in this circumstance I really wish it wasn't. I experiment with the contortion of a smile as I recognise this fact and Sarah, unaware of why I'm trying to smile, beams at my reaction. As she gushes on with her tales, I ponder if this is why people always tell me the same things over and over and over again … maybe they think I don't remember the first five retellings or maybe they've just run out of things to say to me.

'Why don't we go for a walk?' I say when Sarah takes pause to breathe, glancing to the bright blue sky, which is teasing us through the kitchen window.

'We still have the rest of that film to watch and those episodes.'

'We can watch it when we get back. Come on, it's such a nice day,' I point out, a sense of desperation creeping into my gut.

Sarah gets up and collects our empty plates and then places them by the sink to wash later.

'I can't be bothered,' she says, not looking at me.

'All we've done is watch TV … for days,' I say sullenly.

'Why have you got so much energy? You're meant to be sick, remember,' she says jestingly but her words douse my insides with ice.

I can never shake off what they did to me. No matter how many private positive blood tests for Lyme disease I have, no matter how many I can literally hold in my hands, no matter how many years of treatment … the doubt the public doctors hold over my diagnosis … over my very sanity, which they brutally instilled inside me, will never fade.

Her words have stolen what heart I had to argue and instead I compromise when Sarah suggests we bake; even though we baked yesterday and now have more baking than people to eat it. I make sugar-free, wheat-free, yeast-free but, surprisingly, not taste-free brownies made with avocados.

'What are you doing?' Sarah asks sharply, straightening up from putting the trays of baking into the oven.

I look at her and then down at the sink which I'm filling with warm soapy water, confused by her inability to understand the obvious.

'… the dishes,' I say, after a moment's consideration, unsure if I'm being stupid or if she is.

'I'll do it, sit down,' Sarah says, coming towards me to take my place but I hold fast.

'I can wash some dishes,' I say in dismay.

'Of course, you can, but you don't need to,' she tells me, gently pushing against my hip with hers to signal for me to move.

She's worse than Aunt Beth – Joyce leave that, leave this, don't do that, I'll do it later … on and on like I'm incapable of doing anything myself. About a week after Aunt Beth learned about me leaving the house alone, she tackled me on the subject and told me I wasn't allowed to leave the house without her … she quickly lost that battle though when she realised that she had no way of policing it. I stare into the face of my little sister, her freckles standing out strongly on her nose after her holiday in the sun – I remember putting sun cream on that nose as children, I remember putting makeup on it as teenagers … just how much things have changed sinks so deeply inside me that I back away. I don't mean to surrender my stance at the sink, but that's the ultimate result.

I wander dazedly to my dining room and sit on the end of the sofa bed, my eyes trailing around the room and lingering over my box of drugs, the floor that I've had to crawl across like a grown toddler. I look at the stains going up the wall, like faded blood spatters, from when my liquid medication was opened and splattered up the wall. To the sofa bed itself – an inanimate object which evokes such terrible memories of misery. I was tortured on that bed. I was beaten from the inside out, even as my organs shut down and as my brain became as incapable of thought as the pillow it lay on. This room, what I was within it, what I still am ... now disgust me.

I look to the door, hearing Sarah's footsteps coming down the corridor, and I count down, not by seconds but by footsteps, to her appearing in my room ... three ... two ... one

'You coming through?' she asks, her head appearing at the expected time.

'Yeah,' I say meekly.

I follow her to the couch in the sitting room. My eyes look at the TV screen but they're unseeing. My body's too tense, too agitated, my joints complaining from not being used. I hate just sitting here all day doing nothing – why can't she understand that? Why can't she understand or accept that I'm not the person I was even a few months ago. I've spent nearly a decade of my life sitting unable to do anything ... why would I want to waste any more time doing exactly that. Resentment boils inside me ... it's a feeling the sick know too well.

'Why don't we make you up a profile on social media?' Sarah asks, yet again, apparently bored of the film given she's desperate enough to ask when she already knows my answer.

'I don't want one,' I insist.

'It's really good, plus you can find Logan and all your friends.'

I look at her blankly – we both know I don't exactly have

many of those. Sarah pauses upon seeing my expression and quickly changes tactics.

'You could add my friends. You've met them and they all adore you.'

I shake my head; I refuse to concede to my life being sad enough that I have to steal my little sister's friends to make it look like I have my own.

'And you can add all the people you knew in school. You can see what everyone else is up to. Some of them are still in the area – you could get in touch and meet up and you can share pictures and everything,' Sarah lists insistently.

'Why would I want to friend friends who abandoned me when I became ill? And, why would I want to see what they get up to? And what photos am I going to share?' I state bluntly.

I feel cruel for saying it but she won't take no for an answer.

'… Ok,' she says slowly. 'In that case you can go on and laugh at how badly they're all ageing. Here …' she says, pulling her phone out and showing me some of the people I used to be friends with in school who look, rather satisfyingly, far worse than me.

We spend the next thirty minutes laughing at people I used to know and be friends with and it seems so amusing with Sarah next to me, making mocking commentary and pointing things out, that I agree to her setting up an account for me.

'Right come on, let's take Dog out,' I say once the film ends and my account is complete.

'He's fine,' she says with a dismissive hand wave.

'He needs taking out,' I say, looking at Dog, who's raised his head hopefully at the sound of his name.

But Sarah ignores me and simply puts on another film.

'I'll take him,' I say, pulling myself to my feet.

'No, you're not.'

'What?'

'You're not leaving the house on your own – not when I'm in here and in charge.'

'In charge?' I splutter.

'I'm not taking responsibility if something happens because you've gone off on your own.'

'Then come with me,' I suggest.

'No. I don't want to,' she says, obstinately crossing her arms.

'Well, I'm taking Dog out so you can come or you can stay but either way I'm going,' I tell her, standing by the sitting-room door, waiting for her to come with me.

'You're not going,' Sarah orders from the couch.

'I'm not a child Sarah, you can't stop me. I'm not the little sister here.'

'Yeah but essentially you are, aren't you? You can't look after yourself. You can't even make yourself lunch,' Sarah snaps at me.

I stand ... stunned. I want to yell that the only reason I couldn't is because she wouldn't let me, but instead I move numbly to the cupboard and put on my jacket and shoes. I spot Sarah as she heads back into the sitting room as I come out of the kitchen and head to the front door. Once I'm ready I call mutedly to Dog who's already waiting excitedly at the front door. I go to open it but it's locked. My hand automatically reaches to unlock it but my fingers swipe through the air where the key should be. I go to the back door but it's locked and the key is missing from it too. I go back to the sitting room to find Sarah on the couch, studying the screen of her phone.

'Looking for these?' she says smugly, holding up the keys.

'What are you doing?' I demand.

'I told you, you're not leaving the house. I'm not taking responsibility for something happening to you.'

'I'm an adult.'

'No, Joyce, you're not!' Sarah says brutally.

I stare at her and it hits me what that look in her eyes is … it's fear. She's scared of me. She's scared to leave the house with me, never mind me leaving it alone. My own sister is afraid of me. I swallow hard against the roughness in my throat, like sandpaper against a stone, it seems it's not just me who has to relearn how to trust my body. I back away from the sitting room and go to my dining room with Dog eagerly following behind me. I pace back and forth. The coldness of my sadness thawed by the heat which is coursing through me with such velocity that I'm shaking … It feels odd to shake from something other than fatigue – I forgot the two could feel so different. Dog's head follows my movements back and forth, his head tilted in confusion. He makes a rumbling noise as though he's slowly going to grow his voice into a bark but he fades it out into a whine when I glare at him.

Chapter Thirteen

JOYCE – AGE 23

Ok, so it's maybe not the most mature move I've ever made, I decide ten minutes later as I march (or what a healthy person would consider a slow to normal paced walk) down the road with Dog's bushy tail flouncing ahead of me. But I refuse to be turned into a prisoner inside my own prison. I pause on the empty road to cup my knee, which I caught on the wall just beneath my window ledge, the smarting sting forewarning of the graze I suspect I've given myself. I shake my head, both gleeful and bashful. I'm twenty-three and I just climbed out of my own window, like a skulking teenager sneaking out after dark. The twenty-three-year-old in me left a note to say that I've gone for a walk with Dog – although it was no easy feat getting him through the window. A vague sensation of embarrassment and rebellion battles inside me for dominance as I resume my walk. I feel like a ping pong ball, constantly swinging between being an adult and the sixteen-year-old I was when I became housebound. I've no idea which one is me or if I'm both. It's like I'm Jekyll and Hyde, only of less violent extremes.

When I reach the corner, I pull myself up onto the top bar of the gate into the neighbours' fields, my internal burning ebbing away into exhaustion. The cool metal slowly warming under the heat of my body, the sheep lazily grazing in the field before me. I make myself smile as I recall the memory of feeding the lambs at Logan's but somehow the external smile doesn't radiate inwards like I hoped it would. I sit there until Dog's impatient whines pull my mind away from a past life that seemed so simple. Reluctantly, we head home. As I enter the drive, I spot Aunt Beth's car sitting in the driveway. I pause to consider my window but now Aunt Beth is home and the self-imposed prison guard will have been let off duty, there's really no point. Besides, doesn't it defeat the purpose of rebelling against someone if they don't know you've done so?

So, I head to the open back door and enter through the utility into the kitchen. Dog pushes past me to run up to Aunt Beth, who's making dinner. Sarah is sitting at the table. The wide smile playing around her lips, from whatever message her latest boyfriend just sent her, melting off her face like ice held up to a heater when she sees me. There's a long and awkward pause as my presence is registered.

'Nice walk?' Aunt Beth asks, the strain in her voice hinting at how hard she's trying in order to sound casual.

'Very,' I say pointedly, catching sight of my note on the worktop.

I take off my trainers and jacket and set about putting them away as dinner is served. When I return, Sarah is sitting in my usual chair. She looks at me, her head tilted and her eyes narrowed, waiting for me to react. She knows fine well I need that seat, that at this time of night the light from the setting sun is too bright and it burns my eyes. No words are spoken though as I cross the room and sit in the opposite chair. My eyes watering as Aunt Beth places the food before us but I refuse to narrow my eyes against the glaring sunlight.

I don't partake in the dinnertime conversation, which isn't unusual ... Let's face it, what do I have to contribute? My opinion is never sought anyways, besides I'm too busy methodically forcing myself to eat the potato and chicken salad through my nausea to even listen. I shut my eyes for a moment, hunting for some relief, the back of my eyeballs burning.

As soon as I'm finished eating, I get up and leave the room without bothering to wait for Sarah or Aunt Beth to finish their meal. I quietly close the door of my dungeon and stare glumly about my dining room before reluctantly sitting on the sofa bed. I'm slowly learning that there is something worse than being bedbound and that's being able to leave but having nowhere to go.

I gaze at my window, the temptation resurfacing but the weight in my body and the gnawing pain in my limbs is warning me I've done enough today. Instead, I open my laptop and my new social media account instantly springs up. One of the icons is flashing and, when I click on it, its headline tells me I have five accepted friend requests and seven people who have sent me one. I run my finger across my lips to feel the foreign sensation of a smile upon them. The ghost of affection flickering across my eyes as I recognise some of the names who have sent me requests. Maybe I've not been as forgotten as I thought. Maybe the impression I left on the world before I died still exists. An absurd feeling of being accepted and vaguely wanted stirs within me as I click on their profiles and scroll through them. I hungrily absorb the information about their lives and the extraordinary things they have done with them. All the jobs they've worked, their degrees, holiday pictures, how many likes and comments they have on their posts, how the odd picture is captioned with 'the school gang reunited' while faces I once knew so well stare back at me.

I lean forwards, my mind ensnared by the never-ending web of people from my past. Each picture or comment linking to someone else I once knew. I'm stunned by their lives, their relationships. We're the same age yet some of them are married and some are parents. I swallow hard at the sandpaper in my throat. My insides crumpling at the sight of their huge and beautiful lives – the contrast swallowing me whole.

I know I shouldn't but, in the growing darkness, I search on my laptop for the picture of Sarah and me from just before I had to drop out of school. We had just finished doing our makeup for a party and, in the picture, we both look at the camera with our heads tilted together in a tender gesture of affection, our eyes narrowed in mirth, alight with life ... we never knew mine was fading.

Sarah and I were so close, we did everything together and I was always the one she came to. Our lives were so integrated and I paved the way for her to follow me in her own unique way but my path crumbled and she was forced to find her own. I look into the eyes of my little sister, who has now superseded me in every manner possible. She wasn't lying when she said I wasn't an adult; I may have the status in age but in age alone. She's older than me in every other sense. She has matured into an adult while I've reverted back into a child. The world and everyone in it has moved on, advanced, whereas I've become undeveloped, stagnated, my only advancement in life is that I'm alive and right now that doesn't seem to count for much.

I get off the bed and open the window to the crystal-clear sky of summer's night. Pulling myself up onto the thin window ledge, I wedge my body between the frame of the window so that I can stare, unhampered by the glass, up at the sky. My eyes move between the stars, those bright burning dots trapped in darkness. Joy seems as far away as they are. Each day the distance between us grows longer and the harder it is to remember who she was. I would do anything, anything at all, to go back and be me. I just want this to stop, just for a moment, just so I can feel like I can breathe. I'm so very tired of being tired but mostly I'm tired of being scared of the monster living within me.

I try to silence the thoughts that Sarah's words ignited but they whirl around my head like wasps, buzzing around me before boldly stinging me with the words that were spoken during the years of fighting for my illness to be found: 'You don't think it's in her head, do you?' my sister had said. 'Mental barriers which are stopping you from getting better,' Dr Careless's voice whispers viciously. 'Psychological elements!' 'Therapy might be good for you,' Logan's message repeats in my head. 'Are you saying this is all in my head?' I'd asked. 'Yes,' Dr Burk replied.

I hate you. I hate you all … is all I can think as I gasp at the crisp night air, the cavern opening up inside me as I weep into the darkness.

Chapter Fourteen

JOYCE – AGE 24

The challenges of the sick which most take for granted:

- Restaurants – when you have a strange diet the chances are you're going to spend half your time eating things you don't actually want to eat because the thing you do want you can't eat. From sugar in soups to wheat in your chips. They might say they cater to your diet but in reality, they often don't.

- Cars – you see a nice car and think … Oh, I wouldn't mind one of those. I see a nice car and go … Oh, I'd need a forklift to get out of one of those. An average car is nothing short of humiliating for sick people to get out of because they are so low to the ground and any seat with a lip/bucket style seat is nothing short of a nightmare.

- Cinema/theatre – I won't lie, I've not even attempted it … noise, burning bright screen, steps (if you don't want to be sat so close to the screen you feel like you'll snap your neck), seats you need balance, coordination and the ability to squat, twist round and pull down all at the same time, plus tons of people squeezed in beside you. It's a no-go from the start.

- Appointments in general – Ops, after all that planning between you and your carer on what time is best and how you're going to get there, you hear this from the reception desk … 'I'm sorry, you've missed your appointment.' Yup, because in between them telling you the appointment on the phone and you writing it down as they give it to you, your wonderfully diseased brain has decided to muddle the time and date of the appointment for you. The joys of having Lyme brain!

- Hairdresser – most people quite enjoy going for a haircut but for me, with my hypersensitiveness, attending a hairdresser's where they have music playing, hundreds of different chemicals wafting about, hair dryers blasting and people yelling over each other to make inconsequential conversation … Well, I may as well have my head next to a speaker at a rock concert for the screaming weeklong headache I come away with.

I sit, curled up amongst the blankets on my sofa bed. Working my way through a wordsearch, another seemingly pointless exercise that is surprisingly mentally advantageous, when Aunt Beth comes into my room and sits at the end of my bed. She stares into the cold emptiness of the fireplace but says nothing. I watch her for a minute, my pen tapping increasingly loudly against my wordsearch.

'What's wrong?' I ask, eventually, when no explanation for her sudden appearance arises.

'I was talking to Kate, the other night, about her engagement,' Aunt Beth begins hesitantly. 'And she'd like to do something for it. I thought maybe we should have a party here for them.'

I instantly recoil deeper into the cushions behind me.

'I looked at some venues last night but they're too much to hire,' Aunt Beth hastens to add.

I quickly look away, my eyes falling onto the box of drugs which she spends thousands of pounds on to maintain.

'I don't really have time to organise anything either but I was wondering if you would organise it? I know it would mean a lot to Kate …' Aunt Beth continues.

I continue to stare at the box of drugs in the corner of my room. I can't deny, despite everything, how much I owe Kate. She's fallen into the category of being my carer more times than I'd like to recall but the idea of trying to organise something like that when I can hardly manage to buy myself toothpaste …

'What would I need to do?' I ask, reservedly, my pen now still against my wordsearch.

'Well, we have the big gazebo in the garage still … I think it should be ok, so we can put that up. And then all we need is invites to be sent out, decorations, food and drink really,' Aunt Beth says, ticking each item off on her fingers. 'Oh, and music.'

'I don't know any of her friends,' I point out.

'You can invite them on that social … thing. Listen, have a think and let me know,' she says, getting up off my bed and leaving me to ponder the prospect.

I look out the window at the late afternoon sun, debating to myself if I'm being selfish. The idea of having so many people here, all the movement, noise, pressure … even the thought of it makes the serpent of sickness coil in my stomach and my pulse to quicken. I tap the end of my pen against the puzzle book, a twinge of bitterness in my gut, my cousin is getting married and I've never even been on a date. I can't even remember the last time I celebrated something, my eighteenth was spent in bed, my twenty-first was spent on treatment – although I didn't mind not marking it, I don't find pleasure in noting that fact that I'm getting older when I've yet to be young.

I subconsciously rub my leg, recalling when Kate came to visit after my first treatment, how she sat me down in the sitting room and painstakingly shaved my legs for me. It's safe to say that when you can hardly feed yourself, being able to shave is hardly a high priority. At the time, I'd recovered enough to be able to shave my underarms but even that was a strong struggle. She was so tentative, so cautious, so terrified of cutting me and causing me more pain. I remember lying in bed that night and simply running my fingers up and down my legs. The smooth sensation so tantalising that I couldn't stop myself from feeling my own skin – until my frail arms grew too tired to move.

I lean over the side of the sofa bed and pull my laptop out from under it. Opening it, I search for engagement themes and decoration ideas before I can talk myself out of doing so. There're banners, bunting … the usual stuff but then I find a site which has thousands upon thousands of ideas for unusual decorations.

Later that day, I run my suggestions past Aunt Beth while we sit at the kitchen table. She's sceptical at first, worried by how much it will all cost but I explain how I plan to make them … which only increases her scepticism but she agrees to let me order the things I need nonetheless. I spend the rest of the day planning out and ordering all the stuff required. When I go through the online checkout and I'm brought back to the site's homepage, I notice an advert for online studying.

I hesitate, my cursor hovering over the link for more information. I feel a twinge of something like fear as I click on it and I'm taken to their site, my eyes tracing each line I read. By the sounds of it, I could actually study at least one of the subjects I was doing at school before I had to drop out. They have options for doing degrees online but I instantly skip over them, deciding instead to stick within the possibilities of my limits. I never knew there was such a thing as distance learning. The internet was an unreliable commodity before I got ill – you could never depend on not getting the circle of death as it tried to load anything. It seems so obvious to me now, though; we can watch TV through the internet so why couldn't you study through it too? I click to read about the costs, entry requirements, exam details and more. Other than two trips to the local college, for exams, I wouldn't be required to even leave the house.

I sit back a little in my chair, the dull sounds of Aunt Beth bustling about in the utility room an undertone to my silent debate. Could I even keep up with the course load? I consider my withered brain and what it's endured these years. Of being so ill I couldn't remember my aunt's name or even who she was, how I still struggle to speak without word misplacement or to recall simple things.

I was sixteen when I was last in any form of education and, let's face it, I wasn't exactly able to attend much of it. What happens if I have a bad week and fall behind … what's more, what if I fail?

I jump a little as my phone buzzes beside me. I pick it up to find a message from Amy. I have to read the name twice before I can convince myself it's truly from her. I've not heard from her in over a year despite my attempts to keep in contact.

Amy: Hey, long time! I'm home this weekend if you fancy meeting up?

I look up dazedly from my phone, wondering where this sudden desire has come from. A large part of me wants to tell her to jog on but then it's not as though I have a large supply of friends or the ability to replenish them.

Me: Hi, this is a surprise. It's been too long! Sure, I think I should be free. What time and where?

I throw in the 'I should be free' to create the illusion that I actually have a life that requires planning beyond being well enough to leave the house that day. She replies almost instantly.

Amy: Why don't we go for coffee? I'll pick you up. Does Friday work? Say 1pm?

Me … hesitantly: Sure, sounds nice. See you then.

I put my phone down on the table and stare at it for a moment, unsure if it's an instrument of invasion or connection. I turn back to my laptop, my fingers instantly moving to click off the page about the course but that image of myself sitting as I am, a further ten years from now, returns to me. I cautiously click to print off the application form and course information instead. Printing it off doesn't mean I have to fill it out, I remind my racing heart.

'Baby steps,' I whisper to myself.

I return to my party planning, my eyes getting lost in a sea of colour, glitter and excited faces. I seem to be coming to the end of my main search because most of what's coming up now are adverts for party hairstyles. I used to enjoy letting Sarah style my hair. We'd take it in turns when we were getting ready for a party. I subconsciously run my fingers through my long but straggly straw-thin hair. I lost a lot of it during treatment. It never came away in big dramatic clumps, it came away in a habitual loss, countless strands of my hair covering my pillows, my tops, my bed covers – you could run your hand across my bedsheets like a rake and gather it up into a ball with your fingers. Brushing it was gut-wrenching for the horrible sight of how much came away. Washing it was even worse, sitting on a stool with my head over the bath, as Aunt Beth washed it. Watching as my hair came away with the water, clogging the drains in an unsightly tangle, was like watching pieces of myself float away. The stem of loss has slowed and new baby-fine wisps of hair are growing in but it's slow to compensate what's been lost. I smooth my hair out to see how long it is – my fingers finding the ends which stop in a scraggily mess more than half way down my back.

'Aunt Beth?' I say, as she comes back into the kitchen.

'Yes,' she says distractedly, filling the kettle before reaching down to rummage in the cupboard for her thermal mug.

'Can I get my hair cut?'

She pauses, then turns around to look at me. 'I can cut it tonight if you want?'

'I mean, at a hairdresser.'

I watch Aunt Beth inhale a deep breath as she considers it. We've had this discussion before and ruled it out.

'Let me see what I can do,' she says.

Chapter Fifteen

AUNT BETH

This was a stroke of luck, I think happily to myself, as Joyce sits at the kitchen table – her pale hands holding onto the outside of her thighs.

I had completely forgotten, until the other day, that my friend's daughter is studying to be a hairdresser and has been hunting for people to practice on. She eagerly took up the opportunity to come round and it meant that Joyce didn't have to go to a hairdresser. Although, Joyce needed some persuading once she heard her lack of credentials. 'You want me to trust what little's left of my hair to someone who's not qualified?' she'd asked, askance. But, the challenges of going to get her hair cut eventually won her over.

'So, what would you like done? Have you got any styles in mind?' the eager girl, of around eighteen, asks.

'I don't mind. Just cut it however you think might suit,' Joyce says uncertainly, squirming slightly in the kitchen chair.

'Ok …' the girl looks flummoxed before adding jokingly, 'to be honest, I wouldn't ever say that to a hairdresser … you might end up with half your head shaved off.'

She runs her fingers through Joyce's hair … pondering. Joyce flinches a little as the girl's nails rake her scalp. When Joyce was on treatment, her skin became so sensitive that she could barely stand the feel of fabric against it and trying to brush her hair would have her gritting her teeth against the soft bristles; which may as well have been thorns.

'What about making it shorter? Your hair's *really* thin. I'd honestly say making it shorter would make it thicker and there'd be less weight on it, too.'

'Ok,' Joyce agrees.

I stare at her, my mouth opening in disbelief. Did she really just agree to having her hair cut short? She takes over five minutes to decide whether she wants a cup of tea or not! I expected her to protest at such a notion … not agree to it. She's had her hair long since she was nine and staged an inhouse protest in the kitchen about growing it. Of course, her little sister decided to join the revolt too.

'Are you sure?' the girl asks, as I inwardly cringe at the eager gleam in her eyes.

I really hope she knows what she's doing, I think to myself, my hand covering my mouth to stop myself from saying anything.

'Maybe you should decide how short you want to go first,' bursts through my fingers despite myself, as the scissors make an appearance.

'Yeah, good idea!' the hairdresser says.

'Ehh, ok. I guess no shorter than my shoulders,' Joyce decides on a whim.

I can actually feel my intestines knotting with the anticipation of impending doom. I watch the pair interact as the scissors start chopping away long chunks of Joyce's hair, Joyce's lack of social skills becoming alarmingly apparent. I knew it was something she struggled with but seeing it is a whole different thing. I watch the pair of them, both of their faces in competition as to whose can be the most fastidious. It's almost painful, watching the concentration on Joyce's face as she tries to keep up with the words of the hairdresser and as she tries to ingest their meaning. She's so slow to reply that the conversation is confusingly disjointed. After ten minutes, I can see the effort of communicating with this fast-spoken and chipper girl is draining Joyce. Her eyes are growing heavy and her face pale, her back increasingly stooped – which the girl keeps trying to correct, unable to understand why Joyce is being so uncompliant as she starts sinking just moments after being asked to sit up. I knew as soon as I came home that today wasn't a good day for Joyce – I probably should have cancelled her appointment. I try to make an effort to take over the conversation and both of them looked relieved when I do.

When the girl finally hands Joyce the mirror, we both wait with bated breath for her verdict.

'I don't know if I like it,' Joyce says eventually.

I glance in time to see the girl's excited smile slide off her face to be replaced by shock. She gives herself a little shake of the head as though to shake the comment from in one ear and back out the other.

'I think it really suits you. You've done a great job,' I say quickly, trying to cover over Joyce's bluntness. 'Hasn't she done a great job of cutting it, Joyce?'

'Yeah, it's been cut really well,' Joyce says, thankfully picking up on my hint. '… and it feels really smooth now.'

'Really?' she asks, seeking further affirmation.

'Yeah, I … I know I'll really like it once I'm used to it.'

'Oh, honestly, it'll change your life. So much easier to keep,' she tells us earnestly.

Once she leaves, Joyce slops off to the other room while I sweep up hunks of her hair into the dustpan, the long strands clumping together between the bristles of my brush as though they're resisting being moved any further from their owner. I carry the dustpan to the bin and watch as strands of Joyce fall into the depths of the carrier bag inside it.

I head to the sitting room where I know Dog will be waiting impatiently to see who and what has been going on in his kitchen. I pause as I pass the bathroom, though, to see Joyce looking at herself in the mirror. One hand holding onto the sink as if to steady herself and the other clutching the end of a handful of hair.

'Do you not like it?' I ask uncertainly.

She shrugs one shoulder, her eyes not moving from her own reflection.

'No, it's just …' she begins but stops.

'Just what?' I ask gently, after a moment. Even as a child Joyce never told you things freely, she always needed to feel you wanted to hear it before she felt safe to say it.

'I just thought making such a big change would make me feel … something big,' she says, still without looking at me.

'In what way?' I say, stepping into the doorway of the bathroom.

'Different,' she says quietly.

'It *is* a big change; maybe you just need to let yourself catch up with it,' I say, unsure of her meaning.

Four days later, I come home to find Joyce sitting at the kitchen table with her friend Amy. Bits of card, paint, glitter and glue on every surface. It's like I've walked back in time to find the kids and their friends doing an art project together.

'Hi Amy,' I greet, dumping my work bag and jacket in the utility. 'It's nice to see you. How are you?'

'Yeah, good, thanks!' she says brightly, retying her dark hair into a messy bun. 'How are you?'

'I'm good,' I say, so delighted to see her that I can't hide my smile. 'You two look busy.'

'Amy volunteered to help make the decorations for Kate's engagement party,' Joyce tells me, her voice sounding more alight within Amy's company.

'Yeah, Joy showed me all the ideas she had and I had heaps of stuff at my house that we could use for it,' Amy tells me.

'Like the bottles?' I ask, spotting about ten wine bottles sitting on top of newspaper. They seem to have been spray painted gold on the top and covered in glitter at the bottom – the effect is surprisingly classy.

'Mum never takes the bottles to the bank until she can fill the boot!' Amy laughs.

'These look really good,' I admit, surprised by what they've been able to do.

I loiter around the kitchen, taking an exuberantly long time to make myself a mug of tea, just so I can see Joyce with a friend. I sit in the sitting room to sip at my tea, enjoying the background noise of people rather than silence. I can't remember the last time the house was filled with the noise of Joyce and her friends. I know I should leave them to it but as soon as my cup is finished, I go back to the kitchen and faff about in the utility room just so I can be closer to the glow of something good.

With no reason left to loiter, I head upstairs. I sit on my bed, with my laptop on my knee, searching for cooking classes, dance classes, craft classes. I look up the ones my friends have recommended over the years and then I find a few of my own. There's some which catch my eye and I open tab after tab of classes which spark my curiosity. Slowly though, I close each tab. My heart sinking, into my already lead-lined gut, as I realise I work every moment that I'm not too tired to and how the prices would eat into my already thin budget. I don't have the luxury of doing things for me, I remind myself. I shut my laptop and dump it on the bed next to me. I can't tell if I want to cry or scream. I feel like even if I did … no one would hear. I force myself to get up and head downstairs, pausing halfway, suddenly far less enthusiastic to witness and hear the fun being had in the kitchen. With a sigh, I call to Dog before grabbing my jacket from the bottom of the stairs and heading outside. I didn't plan it, but I run … as hard and as fast as I can. The blood coursing round my body, my legs eager to take up an old habit which has slowly died. It's been so long that I forgot the merciful silence its rhythm brings. When I come in, sweating and with tender feet, the house is once more static with stillness.

In the kitchen, Joyce is sitting with one leg pulled up to her chest – her head resting on top of her knee.

'You have a good time with Amy?' I ask breathlessly, hanging my jacket up.

'Yeah,' she remarks shortly.

'It's nice that she came round.'

'Yeah, that brings her number of visits up to one in the last year,' Joyce says stoically.

'I know, but it's good she came round. People are busy and they get caught up in their own lives,' I say, grabbing a glass from the cupboard and filling it with water.

'I know that,' Joyce all but snaps. 'I'm not ungrateful … I …'

I pause to look at her. What must it be like to have people who were your peers now tower over you? To have them come round and tell you about the exciting things happening in their lives when you have next to none?

'Have you had many more replies from the invites you put out?' I ask, trying to distract her. 'We should probably think about getting the gazebo up in the next day or two.'

'Most people are coming,' Joyce says, rubbing her eyes, not sounding entirely pleased by this.

'Why don't you get a nap?' I suggest, immediately regretting my words.

She shakes her head ... like I knew she would, her eyes brimming with tears. She suddenly looks small, defenceless, childlike.

'Did Amy say something that upset you?' I say, my breathing beginning to steady.

Joyce shakes her head again.

'Everyone has a life,' she splutters. 'Everyone has someone.'

'I know,' I say sadly, going over to stand beside her and pulling her into my side. 'I know.'

Chapter Sixteen

LOGAN – AGE 24

I meander up the drive and around the side of the cottage, which is lined with lanterns and fairy lights, pausing when I spot Joy sitting on the wall. Her hair has been cut short and she wears a fitted dress … somehow the combination is oddly jarring. I'm too used to her being in pyjamas or baggy clothes but, as I near her, I struggle to keep the goofy smile I can feel creeping across my face at bay. Joy is just Joy. I don't really think of her as anything other than that but seeing her now reminds me she's so much more. I inwardly chuckle, spotting a bottle of something suspiciously alcoholic in her hands.

'You know, people who drink alone get a bad reputation?' I laugh, the sound of my voice making her look around.

'Hey,' she exclaims with a smile, watching as I come out of the shadows and into the full light of the lanterns.

She lets herself slip down from the wall and throws her arms around me. I hug her back, laughing at her exuberance.

'I'm so glad you're here,' she says happily into my ear.

'I said I would come,' I say cheerfully.

'I know. You want some?' she says, pulling away from me and holding out the bottle.

I take it from her and take a sip, the cool liquid bubbling

against the roof of my mouth and against my tongue. We head to the wall and sit on it, passing the bottle of prosecco between us.

'So why aren't you with everyone else?' I ask.

She shrugs.

'It was just getting a bit much,' Joy tells me, taking a gulp before handing me the bottle.

'Why?' I ask, watching her closely, the fairy lights and lanterns shining off her eyes.

'Just all the couples and mushy games and stories of first dates,' she explains, her voice taking on the dramatic tones of the tipsy. 'You know, I remember Kate picking her nose and eating it as a kid and yet she's the one who's engaged. I'm happy for her, it's just, she has this fancy job and life and I'm...well, I'm twenty-four, still living at home, have no job, no education and I've never even been on a date.'

'Yeah, but you could easily get a date. Look at you, you scrub up nicely when you're not in pyjamas,' I retort jokingly.

'Ha, thanks,' she tells me, looking down at her dress, swaying a little on the wall as she does so.

'I'll take you on a date,' I promise, handing her back the last of the bottle. 'We'll go somewhere really fancy. I'll even bring you your favourite flowers when I come to pick you up. I'll take you for a nice meal and once I've eaten all my food, I'll have the rest of your food because you're always full after a bite of chicken and half a potato,' I joke, my smile growing at the laughter on her lips. 'We'll have to get a taxi home because I'll be too bloated to fit behind the steering wheel but ... it'll be magical.'

'Sounds like quite the date. Only you missed out the dancing ... there has to be dancing.'

'Oh, well we do that first so we have an appetite for dinner,'

I tell her. 'So, Joyce Jack, will you let me be the first man to take you on a date?'

'You really want to take me on a date?' she asks sceptically, the fairy lights behind her dimming before bursting back into life.

'Course,' I assure. 'Right, come on, let's join the rest.'

'Do we have to?' she asks, twisting round to balance the empty bottle on the wall behind her.

'Think on it this way, you and I have probably been friends longer than those couples have known each other. We can easily beat them at those games. Come one, let's put them to shame.'

She smiles and slips off the wall. I hold out my hand for her to take, her fingers like ice within mine. We head towards the gazebo but before we can reach it loud music begins to blare from within. I watch Joy remove something from inside her bra and fit it into her ears – I figure it must be something to help with her sensitive hearing. I hold my arm up so that she can twirl under it as we enter under the canvas flaps. The busy gazebo is filled with fairy lights; a mishmash of chairs surrounding tables with gold painted and glittered bottles with flowers or feathers sticking out the top; there's a small table dedicated just to sweets; a photo-booth corner with inflatable props; one entire wall is lined with fine white fishing wire, in the centre of which is a photo of Kate and her partner and all around it people have pinned pictures of them together – I smile, now understanding the PS at the bottom of the invitation to take your favourite picture of the couple with you. I jump a little in surprise as Sarah appears from behind me.

'Hi, you having fun?' I shout over the music, as the three of us dance together.

'Yeah, so glad we were allowed to take some friends,' Sarah

tells me, pulling a face that's not dissimilar to Joy's when I first arrived. 'I'm going to get Kate,' she calls excitedly.

Sarah disappears into the crowd as the next song comes on. I burst out laughing as everyone starts jumping up and down together and yelling the words into the air around us. I grab Joy again and spin her round, her laughter unhampered and so full of freedom that I don't want it to stop. Sarah appears with Beth, Kate and her partner - who have both been dressed up in sashes and crowns.

'So good to see you, Logan,' Kate says, leaning over to give me a brief hug.

'Congratulations,' I yell, over the loud singing around us.

The six of us dance about like loons. I watch as Joy's movements grow shorter, her arm gestures less exuberant and as her breathing becomes laboured, but her eyes are alight in a way they've not been since school.

'Wh-what happened?' I try to say, although I suspect my words have formed nothing more than a grunt.

I drag my eyes open. The morning light is filtered through a haze of streaks, like my eyeballs have hundreds of hairline fractures. I moan groggily, opening my mouth and taking a deep breath in, choking as I inhale a mouthful of hair. I sit up, shaking Joy's hair off my face as I do so. I look to the left of me to see Joy sound asleep next to me with Dog and Sarah on the other side. I lie back down, my head pulsating unpleasantly. When I wake up next, Joy, her little sister and three of Sarah's friends are all squished onto various parts of the sofa bed with us, the TV playing in the background.

'How did I drink so much and still wake up feeling like I'm

dying of dehydration?' I moan, rubbing my forehead.

'You how drinking works right?' scorns one of Sarah's friends, who looks like he's still in high school.

'Shooo, the adults are talking,' I tell him, making the rest laugh.

'Are you hungover?' I ask Joy pathetically, somewhat hoping that she is.

'I'm always hungover,' she tells me, the gleam in her eyes showing her amusement at my state of suffering.

'All right, Miss Hardcore,' I tell her, rubbing my forehead, which feels like it's been cleaved in two.

'Seriously?' the teenager asks, removing his eyes from the TV to look at her.

'No,' Joy says incredulously.

'I know what you mean,' I say, nudging her.

When Joy was diagnosed with Lyme disease, I did a bit of reading; one of the things which came up from the patients' description was that, even on a good day, it felt like you've been hit by a truck while having the worst hangover and flu of your life. A part of me wonders if she could even tell the difference between a hangover and her disease?

'Can I just lie on you a minute?' I ask her.

'Yeah,' she says happily, moving her arm so I can shift my head to rest on her lap.

'Oh, is that bacon?' I ask ten minutes later, sitting up again, as Beth walks in holding a tray so large that she has to walk through the door sideways.

'I thought you might be hungry,' she says brightly.

'Ahh, amazing,' Sarah says appreciatively, as everyone who had previously been half asleep suddenly sits up like meerkats.

'The one on the separate plate is for you, Joy,' Beth says, as limbs are pulled up to chests to clear a path for the miraculous miracle which is bacon sandwiches.

I quickly inspect Joy's sandwich which is passed to me to pass to her, I presume it's made of some special bread. I pass her the plate before gleefully taking the sandwich which is handed to me.

'Beth, this is the best thing I've ever tasted,' I tell her, through a mouthful of food.

'There's plenty more,' she says happily, standing in the doorway, watching everyone's eager reactions. 'Anyone want tea or coffee?'

I wait patiently for my turn to give my beverage order and ten minutes later, like the saint of sandwiches, Beth is back with a tray of mugs and yet more bacon sandwiches.

'Thank you!' I say gratefully to Beth, as she hands me another sandwich with my mug. 'We'll help clean everything up after this.'

'There's no rush – enjoy!' Beth tells us, lingering contently in the doorway to watch.

'Like old times,' Joy says quietly, nudging me cheerfully.

'Yeah, it is,' I say contently, finally able to name the feeling I've had since I woke up … It's an odd but also comforting sense of nostalgia.

Waking up in this cottage, hungover, in a bed with more people than space, with Beth in her element as host to a full house of people and Joy showing a genuine hint of happiness … it really is like old times, I think with a smile, as I take another bite.

After another episode of some dumb programme the teenagers like, I decide it's time to rally the troops.

'Right, come on, we better help Beth,' I instruct, despite the desire to curl into a ball.

'Yeah,' Sarah agrees half-heartedly, scraping her hair into a tangled bun.

I sluggishly clamber out of the warmth of the sofa bed after Sarah, as everyone follows suit. I head to the door, the last to do so but I pause at the threshold to see if Joy's following behind me. I open my mouth to make a joke about her trying to skive off cleaning up but my mouth closes tightly as I see her clutching onto the ledge of the fireplace.

'You ok?' I ask anxiously.

'Yeah … of course,' she says dismissively.

I move out into the hall and then wait for her to join me. I watch as she finally appears in the doorway, her body instantly seeking out the door frame to lean against, her hands clinging onto it. It's like someone's pulled the plug on her body. I can almost see her energy circling downward, her body shrinking as the energy drains out of her, her pale skin standing out in stark contrast against her hair and the dark wood of the door frame. I stare at the melting figure, which was full of life just moments before, the swiftness of her digression making my insides clamp with dismay.

Joy stares at the floor, trying to regain her breath, her body shifting slightly as though testing if she can go any further, her unwillingness to give in almost pulpable. I stare at her, not knowing what to say, not wanting to make her feel weak by suggesting she goes back to bed but feeling weak myself for not knowing how to help her.

'I think … I should stay in bed,' she utters so quietly that I'm not convinced I've imagined it.

'Ok,' I say, my voice coming out in little more than a whisper.

She shuffles around and grabs onto the door handle for stability as she takes small and faltering steps back into her room. I take a step forwards, my hand automatically reaching out to help her but something stops me from stepping closer. I stand in the hall, alone, powerless and utterly useless to her. How the heck does she live like this, never knowing one moment to the next when everything that's holding her upright is going to crumble inside her? I swallow hard against the lump building in my throat as memories of her dancing last night fill my mind. Her body moving, seemingly so freely. Her smiling. Her laughing. Her joy. Gone.

I slowly head down the hall and out to the gazebo where I can do something to help … even if it's by cleaning up the evidence of Joy's moment of joy.

Chapter Seventeen

JOYCE – AGE 24

The top things the sick fake:
- We fake being well.
- We fake being happy.
- We fake we're not in pain.
- We fake we don't need help.
- We fake we're not exhausted.
- We fake that we're coping.
- We fake we don't feel lonely.
- We fake we don't mind being left out because you won't make adjustments to make it manageable for us.

Why?
- We fake in order for you to feel more comfortable around us.
- Mostly, we fake in the hope that one day it won't need to be faked.

I hate how quickly the world changes. I can't keep up. Autumn, in all its colourful splendour, came and went. The vividness of the leaves rendered into the bleakness of winter. Aunt Beth always complains about how horrible the weather is but to me it's like living the seasons anew. The icy air nipping my face and cracking my lips as I walk Dog, the ice under my feet, the colours seen in person rather than through a grubby window are still a novelty to me.

I glance out the window before continuing to scroll to the bottom of my laptop screen. When I reach the bottom of the page, I give up and shut the lid. It's a fantasy anyway, I tell myself with a heavy sigh. Every so often I check online to see what part-time jobs are going but then, every time I see something which might suit me, I remember how quickly I became ill after Kate's party. It's one thing doing cleaning or gardening at home, but the reality is I couldn't manage at another person's pace. I did fill out the application for my course though and I was accepted onto it the other day. It starts after summer. That's something … isn't it?

'Shall we go for a walk?' I suggest to Dog, who's lying on the floor next to me. He looks at me without lifting his head. 'You could show a bit of enthusiasm.'

I watch him, assessing his ageing body. It scares me to see his age slowly creeping in. I hate that as I'm becoming more active, he's becoming less so. I've missed the best years of his life and, because of my illness, so has he.

I sigh again. The lights on the Christmas tree twinkle away in the reflection of the glass against the darkening world outside of the sitting room window. Christmas is only a day away and yet its festive spirit doesn't seem to have arrived at the cottage yet. The tree is up, there's lights on the banister, there's even a gingerbread house going stale in the hall but none of it makes it feel like Christmas. I try to be merry and bright for Aunt Beth but the more I fake it on the outside, the darker it feels on the inside. I glance to the coffee table as my phone makes a pinging noise. I reach for it and read the words on the screen.

Logan: Guess who's just got home for Christmas! We're all going to meet for a few drinks at the Bankers Bar tonight if you want to come? I can pick you up on the way.

I stare suspiciously at the word 'we' for a moment before typing my reply.

Me: Who's we?

Logan: The old group.

I bite the inside of my cheeks, my eyes fixed on the screen. I've not seen most of the old group from school since I *was* in school.

Logan: Be really good if you could come!

My automatic response is to say no. I even type it as a reply but I pause as the thought strikes me … I'm twenty-four and I've never even been to a pub. I'm not sure I'm ready to see everyone, though. I sigh in frustration, blowing out my cheeks and then pinching my lips together in consternation, a thousand and one scenarios going through my head as I sit there with two sides of myself fighting the other.

Logan: I'll pick you up at 7 – be ready.

'My silence wasn't a yes,' I say desperately to my phone.

Me: I'm not sure if I can come yet.

Ten minutes later, there's still no reply. I glare at the TV screen, having resigned myself to not going. I'll just have to tell him that when he arrives. I try to focus on the TV as my mind goes to and fro, but I can't help checking the clock. I keep thinking of all the nights out we had as teenagers, of all the laughter and nonsense, of the freedom of simply being, of all the memories. Don't you want to have those kinds of memories again? I hug my ribs as I think of all the nights when I first became ill, when I was trapped in bed unable to leave it; crying because I knew while my insides were screaming from pain, that at that very moment my friends were screaming with joy. All the things I've missed. All the things I'll miss again. While I flick through each dull mundane channel, a voice keeps whispering in my ear that I've missed enough. I'm not stupid, I know my opportunities are limited. One like this might not come for another year ... if at all.

Just get ready, I tell myself, then if you decide to go you at least can. I head to my dining room and pull open my drawers to assess what I have to wear – unsure of the dress code. I've seen on TV the two extremes of dress that people wear for a night out but somehow it doesn't seem appropriate for either. I rummage, my anxiety growing with each item I disregard as I become increasingly aware that all my clothes are old, misshapen and faded. I'd never really noticed before but, looking at them now, I'm embarrassed to be seen in them.

I pull on a pair of Sarah's old jeans she left me, a top and my pre-illness boots as the gremlins in my stomach gnaw away at me. I head down the hall to the kitchen, savouring the official sounding clipping noise of my steps. I quickly put Dog out the back door and hasten to write a note to Aunt Beth to say where I've gone.

I stare at the words for a moment and then whisper them, feeling the sensation of the words upon my lips. I leave the note propped up against the kettle before letting Dog back in.

'Be good,' I say gently to Dog, giving him a hug as a car turns into the drive.

We used to drive past the ancient, almost Tudor-like pub every day on the way to school. It sits on the edge of the village, neither a part of it nor separate from it. I've always wondered what it's like inside. As we park and head out of the car, the cacophony of voices from within builds and grows with every step we take towards it. I clutch the outside of my thighs, the gremlins inside me taking deeper and deeper bites of my gut. Logan opens the door and the noise inside hits me like a gust of wind, the unexpected force snatching my breath.

Hesitantly, I follow Logan inside, feeling my stomach clench as my gaze falls on the nearby table where my past friends sit in a big group. I instantly recognise Connor, Rebecca, Amy and Jamie, who are all sitting together … just like old times. I glance over faces only vaguely known to me until my eyes lock onto Stephen. I hold him in my gaze, as he talks exuberantly to the others at the table. I force myself to look away – my gremlins turned to ice.

'Is that Kenny?' I ask Logan, numbly following his lead to the bar.

There are so many faces I know. Some altered by time, others almost unrecognisable, some almost the same as the day we left school. It's strange to see who's blossomed into beauty and who's wilted and withered. Those who had such high statuses for being elite in looks fading into nothing … I wonder if they'll think the same of me?

'Yeah, he moved back a year or so ago. What do you want to drink?' he asks.

'What? Oh, sorry,' I say, my brain slow to catch up.

I stare at the rows of bottles on the shelves behind the bar – all different shapes and sizes, their contents in different shades of pink, orange, green, brown, red and, of course, clear. The only drink I can really remember having was exceedingly cheap vodka, which tasted like how chemical cleaner smells. I stare at the dizzying array of options, struggling to take any of them in – never mind pick one out.

'What are you having?'

'Probably a beer,' Logan tells me unhelpfully. 'Do you want a spirit?'

'I don't know what that is,' I confess, as I squeeze in closer to the bar to let a group of guys past.

He looks at me, bafflement in his eyes until it seems to dawn on him and he says with growing comprehension, 'You've not been to a bar before, have you? Ok, ehh, why don't you get a vodka and coke?'

'I'm not sure I should really break both the alcohol and sugar ban on the same night,' I point out.

'Ok, gin and tonic it is,' he decides for me. 'Will you order? I've been needing the bathroom since before we left. Just order that one.'

Logan points to the beer tap three along from me and disappears before I can protest. I watch as he pauses by Stephen's table and says hello before carrying on to wherever the toilets are hidden. I tense as Stephen's eyes turn to me – his expression instantly lighting up in amazement. He stands up so quickly that the other occupants of the table have to snatch at his drink to prevent it from spilling.

'Joy!' he beams, racing towards me.

I glance around but there's nowhere to hide. Fake it till you feel it, I decide there and then. I make myself mirror his smile.

'Hi,' I say as brightly as I can.

'Look at you, come here,' he says eagerly, his long arms wrapping themselves around me – holding me fast against his tall frame.

It takes me a moment to react but slowly my arms reach up to hug the boy, correction, the man, who was once my best friend.

'I can't believe it's you. It's so good to see you. How are you?' he asks, pulling away.

It's almost shocking how little he's changed. He's still just as tall and seemingly as athletic. Although, I can see the stumps of stubble which were never there before and his dark hair's almost black now. I remember the girls in school having a debate over who had the nicest eyes ... Logan or Stephen. Logan always used to win but now I'm not so sure.

'Yeah, good thanks. How are you?'

'Good. I can't believe you're here. I've not seen you in ...'

'Eight years,' I pointedly fill in for him.

'Yeah, must be,' he says, awkwardly clutching the back of his neck as the barman finally comes over. 'What you having?'

'Gin and tonic and Logan was getting a ... erm,' I stutter, before pointing to the one he wanted.

'I'll get these,' Stephen instantly offers.

'Oh ... Ok, I'll get the next one.' The line I've heard so often in movies slips so easily from my lips it's as though I've said it a thousand times before.

'So, what have you been up to?' Stephen asks.

'I ... ehh ...' I stammer but the barman thankfully cuts us off by putting the machine next to Stephen so he can pay.

Stephen insists on me waiting for Logan at the table who, as it turns out, is standing two tables away immersed in an animated conversation with another group.

Everyone greets me like a long-lost friend ... which, I suppose, I am. It's as though I've come back from being away on a near decade-long holiday and they can't believe I'm really home. There are some people I'm genuinely pleased to see again and who seem to feel the same, their genuineness making those who use their enthusiasm as a front all the more obvious, while others use it to cover their awkwardness. Logan tries to stay beside me as much as possible but he's forever speaking to someone or being called over to another table. I sit, awkward and alone, unsure of how to make conversation. To give Stephen his due, he involves me in what's being said, trying to pull me out of myself when I'm struggling to do so but a lot of the things they speak of are foreign to me – terms and technology, fads and fashions I know nothing about. My thoughts, feelings, opinions and views are dated ... antiquated and unsophisticated. I'm a child hanging out with the adults. I don't know where someone like me can fit in.

I listen to them chat, surprised by the variety in their jobs. A lot of them come over to sit beside me to chat one-on-one. It's strange how many of them, who everyone had such high expectations of in school, have achieved so little and yet those who teachers paid little attention to have superseded them. You see it in their reaction when you ask what they do, their justification for not being further on in life than they themselves had hoped for ... it's something I recognise within myself. At least I have a valid excuse for my life not amounting to anything. The reaction I get to my life's achievement of being alive is a mix of pity, embarrassment, shock, empathy and admiration ... the latter I never saw coming. At least I now have my course to abate my shame ... I don't correct them when they presume it's a degree. Everyone says how good I look, that they had no idea how sick I was or that they knew I'd been ill but never knew how badly. They all say we'll need to hang out sometime ... I smell bullshit but I play along.

I chat to Jessica for a while, a girl I sat beside every day for nearly six years and who frequently used to stay at mine: another friend who forsook me. I watch her chat about her work and the flat she's saving up to buy with her partner, only partly listening, my eyes drawn instead to her hand gestures. I never realise until now that I don't ever use any. I guess I didn't have anyone to use them with but it's more likely that all unnecessary expenditures of energy were subconsciously binned. I start paying attention to people's movements. The tilts of their head, their bouncing nods, drummed fingers and altering tones. I store them in my mind, try them on with the next person I speak to and discard the ones which don't feel natural. It's like playing at dress up only for gesture and phrases and tones of voice.

I lose track of how many gin and tonics I have. I take each sip like it's medicine, numbing me from the habitual humiliation of having to constantly explain how I am, where I've been all this time, what I've been up to, what Lyme disease is, how it affects me. On and on and on it goes. Constantly repeating myself to people who were once my closest friends. I take each sip because it makes those around me more bearable. I sip again because it makes the world easier to be a part of. I finish each glass because it makes it fun. It brings the Joy out of Joyce and soon the night becomes more than just bearable.

Chapter Eighteen

BETH

I stand in the middle of the kitchen, staring at the note in my hand. I glance down at Dog, who's looking up at me with the guilty eyes of a co-conspirator. I reread the scant words of 'Gone to the pub with Logan' once more. It doesn't state when she went, how long she'll be, how she's getting back just ... simply, gone to the pub. Because, after all, that's the normal thing for a chronically sick girl, with a compromised immune system, to do. She's not even supposed to drink alcohol. For all I know she went at 11am this morning and is currently passed out under a table.

I don't know if Joyce has ever been to a pub before. I think of her in the café, panicking over what to order off the menu, of her struggling to hold a conversation with the hairdresser, of her becoming overwhelmed on the street by the small number of people walking past her. How on earth will she cope with being in a pub full of people?

I wrap my arm around my waist, feeling strangely abandoned. My status as superfluous is hurtling towards me faster than I'm ready for. It's all happening too fast. Most parents have almost an entire decade to prepare for their teenager to become an adult but Joyce has gone from being as dependant on me as a newborn into an encroaching adult within the space of two years. Her life is starting to move beyond mine. I'm now the one who is being left behind. I cross my arms as my eyes skim over her note again, isn't this what I always wanted? Isn't this what we've been working towards? Shouldn't I be jubilant? I need to at least try to be, I decide.

I take my phone out from my pocket and type a message.

Me: Just got your note. Let me know if you need picked up …

I pause, struggling to type what I know I must.

I add: … have a good time.

I check my phone's not on silent and then make dinner – ensuring I make enough for Joyce if she's hungry when she gets back. Then I clean up. I watch TV, I hoover. I take Dog for a walk. Finally, I pace up and down the hall. Over and over again. I check my phone again – deluding myself into believing that I heard it beep. All these years I've longed to be in my own home, in my own company and never once, in all my longing and dreaming, was it this stressful. At least before, all the realms of possible calamities were limited to what could realistically happen to Joyce within the confines of the cottage but this … this is a recipe to my own personal mental breakdown. My fingers itch at an almost overpowering longing to call her. I have to keep reminding myself that she's with Logan and that Logan will keep her safe.

Nonetheless, I keep my shoes on and my car keys near me at all times in case I need to make an emergency dash to the car. By the time I get the message I've been waiting for, asking me if I wouldn't mind picking her up, I've already collapsed on the couch having worked myself into a state of exhaustion. Nonetheless, I heave myself up to head out.

'How was your night?' I ask grudgingly, as I pull away from

the pub with Joyce and Logan in the back.

'Good,' Joyce's enlivened voice calls from the back.

I glance in the rear-view mirror, the word 'good' taking me by surprise. Nothing is ever good. With Joyce, it's always fine … ok at best. As I drive, I try to ignore the alcohol induced fumes coming from the back but it's harder to ignore their conversation – conducted at a far louder volume than is necessary. Joyce's tinnitus will be fun for her tomorrow, I think to myself. I don't pay much attention to what they're saying, only to the hum of their elated tones and the lyrical sound of their laughter. In the darkness of the driver's seat, I feel myself starting to smile at the infectiousness of their happiness.

Chapter Nineteen

JOYCE – AGE 24

There's a reason rates of depression increase during the holidays. There's a reason I dread them:

- Christmas – a celebration of friends and family. Well, I don't exactly have many of either. Besides, hearing and seeing on TV all the excitement and fun everyone else is having, while I'm in a bucketload of pain, isn't exactly my idea of festivity.
- Birthdays – the day you came out of someone's uterus. First, I really don't need reminding that I'm getting older; death and I are already well acquainted, thank you.
- New Year – says what it is on the tin. Beyond still being alive, I haven't achieved much within the last year … or pretty much the last ten … I don't need that fact shoved in my face more than it already is, thanks.

Oddly enough though, this year I don't resent the happy people on TV or the tales of Sarah and Kate's Christmas nights out with work and uni friends. I don't find their happiness induces sadness. I don't even fear the impending New Year.

Perhaps it's because in the days after my pub excursion, I find myself in a swirl of social popularity. My friend requests have taken a steep incline from the people I reunited with at the pub and, from us linking as friends, other people I used to know have found me too. It was the message from Stephen inviting me to his New Year party that really took me by surprise though. It's a strange kind of dilemma I find myself in now: on the one the hand, these people abandoned me when I needed them the most and on the other hand, they're my ticket to regaining the life I've lost. When I shared this notion on Boxing Day with Aunt Beth, Sarah, Kate and her partner, who all had arrived late on Christmas Eve to find me more than a little merry, Aunt Beth took their side.

'They were very young,' she said, spooning sprouts onto her plate.

'So was I,' I point out.

'Well,' Aunt Beth flustered, attempting to keep her rolling sprouts on her plate as they make a dash to freedom. 'They've probably grown up a lot since then.'

'Maybe you should give then another chance,' Sarah suggested, a fork full of dry turkey on route to her mouth.

And, that's why I now find myself standing in a room full of people who were years above and below me at school – along with a mix of strangers whose connection to Stephen I'm completely ignorant off. So far, I've played five games of beer pong (turns out the rules are far simpler than I expected) and, amazingly, I've won four out of five rounds. I've continued my rendition of repetition on how I am, where I have been all this time and what's new with me, all while resisting the urge to point out that *this is* what's new to me! And now I'm sitting in the large lounge with a girl, who I suspect I went to school with but who I have absolutely no recollection of, as she waffles on about complete nonsense.

'You should just do it, like travel the world,' she tells me dreamily, attempting to take another swig from her glass and just about upending it over us.

'… Don't have the money,' I say quickly, realising she's expecting a response.

'Ahh, that's the problem,' she says, sorrowfully.

'What's a problem?' comes a familiar voice.

'Logan,' I cry, desperately relieved to see him approaching us.

'She doesn't have money to trun-travel,' the girl explains.

'Having fun, Cass?' Logan laughs.

'Yeah, she is so nice by the way. Like, I want to adopt her and go travelling with her but she has no money to go travelling,' Cass says, slurring towards the end.

'Why don't you do a TravelerStay?' Logan suggests to me, squeezing onto the end of the couch beside Cass, who automatically droops her head on his shoulder.

'What's that?' I ask, taking a sip from my glass.

'It's a site. You sign up and you just …' Logan pauses as he struggles to find the words. I smile as I realise he's actually quite drunk. Maybe I am as well because I can't stop my mouth from turning upwards. 'Make a profile and sign up to it and then you can go all over the world for free basically. You can go to hostels or farms or whatever and all you do is a couple hours work a day. And, you get your food and a bed for free and the rest of the time is yours to sightsee or sunbathe or whatever – whatever you want.'

'So … what, you just pay for your flights?' I ask, taking another sip and clipping my teeth off the glass instead.

Maybe I *am* a little drunk … having said that, my spatial awareness is so poor that I often do that sober.

'Yup.'

'I want to do that!' I say, keenly. 'Wait, we should do it together!'

Logan thinks for a moment before shouting towards the kitchen, 'Stephen, where's your laptop?'

'On the back unit. Please don't break it,' he calls back from the kitchen.

I fetch the laptop for Logan, who is pinned to the couch by the half unconscious Cass.

'What are you guys up to?' Stephen asks, coming to join us on the already cramped couch.

'Signing up to TravelerStay ... including you,' Logan adds over the cheers of whoever has just won at beer pong, glancing over to Stephen.

I try to correct my face as I feel myself grimace. I can't bring myself to look but I'm painfully aware of Stephen's glance towards me.

'Ehh, no, it's all right. You and Joy do it,' he says, to my great relief.

'Ah, come on, it'll be like old times,' Logan says, dismissing Stephen's comment as he types away on the laptop.

'Honestly, I'm not fussed,' he says, looking round towards where a loud bang followed by a clamour of raucous laughter emanates from. 'Back in a sec.'

Before long, all three accounts are set up.

'I said not to make me one,' Stephen states, re-joining us at the end of the couch.

Logan ignores him and hands me the laptop so I can have a look at my profile. I rub my bottom lip with my fingers as I read his words. He's given me far more attributes than I would have given myself.

'Do you think I need to put a bit in about my ... ehh, Lyme?' I ponder, forgetting the name of my own illness for a moment.

I squint a little as I try to read the words, which keep moving about the page.

'No one will want you if you tell them that,' Cass pipes up.

'Harsh,' I laugh.

'I think you should tell them,' Stephen states.

I look to Logan.

'I wouldn't,' he says, with a shake of his head.

'You can't not tell them,' Stephen says earnestly.

'Ok, ok,' Logan says, but I note he doesn't change anything.

We spend the next hour before we're due to head into town looking through all the different host profiles and all the things we could do. There are so many options that I suggest narrowing it down to hostels. In my drunkenness, I like the idea of being around people.

Despite the booze, I start getting tense in the taxi, my chest getting tighter and tighter as we leave the darkness of the countryside behind us and we're submerged in the lights of the city up ahead, everyone's exuberantly loud voices bounce off the van's interior – hitting me like stray bullets. I clutch onto the outside of my thighs, glancing at Logan, who's in the row of seats in front of me, telling myself there's nothing to be scared of. Thousands of people go to clubs and nothing bad happens to them. What you've seen on TV isn't a true representation, I remind myself. It's not fear you feel, it's excitement, it's an adventure, I tell myself as we come to a stop outside of a packed pub.

I clamber out of the taxi and follow our group inside, grateful, that we get to skip the queue thanks to Stephen knowing the bouncers. I'm not sure my aching back and knees could manage the long wait in the cold otherwise. Everyone has their ID out and ready to be checked but I have to hunt in my bag for mine, my fingers fumbling in the unexpectedness of it all.

Once admitted, we're instantly caught in the swell of music and dragged into a tide of people. I resist the urge to clutch my ears as the pressure of the noise feels like my skull might implode. I follow everyone as they head to the bar, my eyes locked onto those I'm with – scared to lose them in the crowd. My arms are jostled by those around me and I nearly drop the musician's earplugs, which Aunt Beth bought for me for Kate's engagement party, that I've just retrieved from inside my bag. Once inserted, the tones instantly become more bearable.

'You ok?' Logan asks, as I lean up against the bar, holding onto it like it's an anchor.

'Yeah,' I say, looking around at all the people I came out with and trying desperately to memorise their faces and what they're wearing in case I lose them.

'I'm going to go to the bathroom,' Jessica informs us.

'I'll come too,' I say, deciding to take my opportunity while it's there.

I forgot women went to the bathroom in packs. I never understood the desire until now. It's masqueraded as sociability but in truth it's a primal instinct for safety.

Jessica takes my hand and leads me towards the bathrooms. They're packed, hot, noisy and a hazard for women stumbling in heels that I wouldn't even attempt to put on.

'Wait for me, won't you?' Jessica asks fervently, as we locate two empty stalls.

'Yeah, of course,' I say, glad that she's said it before I did.

I push open the door and lock it behind me. The tiled floor littered with stray pieces of toilet roll and litter, an empty glass propped up on the toilet-roll dispenser to compliment the lipstick next to it. I take a deep breath and rest my head against the back of the cubicle door. Here, in my makeshift divider from the world, I try to keep myself together, to keep myself in proportion to the world around me. You can do this, I tell myself as my breathing strains against the invisible bands tightening around my chest. This is what you wanted, to go on nights out, to have fun, to laugh … to be free. So why don't I feel it? Take a breath, take a step. One step. One breath. One step. One breath—

'Hey, excuse me, can you pass me some loo roll,' asks a woman on my left, her hand appearing expectantly between the gap of my cubical wall and the floor.

I know it's the booze but still, I smile incredulously. What on earth has happened to my life. Who'd have thought, even six months ago, I'd be here now. I shake my groggy head, trying to focus on where I am now.

'Yes!' I proclaim to my invisible toilet attempt-ee.

I pull a wad out and hand it to her.

'Thanks,' she says gratefully.

One step. One breath. One step. One breath. I quickly go to the bathroom and head out to wash my hands amidst a crowd of ladies who are chatting and reapplying makeup at the sinks. When Jessica finally appears, we head back out to meet everyone else.

'Here's your drink. I think she might have given us all doubles so just watch,' Logan says, handing me a glass, before whispering to me, 'Cass's on water but don't tell her.'

'Oh, I love this song, come on,' Jessica shouts over the music, grabbing my hand again and pulling at me to follow her.

I let Jessica drag me through the torrent of moving people, the world swirling around me as we push our way through the pub, along a dark corridor and into the adjoining club. I snatch glances at people as we move amongst them, my lips smiling at the excitement of the people around us. At the elation of seeing other people, hugging and laughing with such unhampered happiness.

Jessica grabs my other hand as we reach the dancefloor, the music vibrating through my muscles. I sway awkwardly, looking around to see what everyone else is doing and trying to replicate them. After a moment, I close my eyes and just let myself and the booze circulating my system feel the music and, before I know it, I'm dancing like I've never not. Jessica and I dance up against each other and I tip my head back laughing, the lights and shadows of everyone moving swishing around me.

'Having fun?' Stephen asks over the music, finally finding us.

'Yeah but why are all the men here so old and creepy?' I ask, glancing around us again.

'Old …' he says, looking around. 'They're the same age as us. Well, except those ones. They're fresh out of the pram.'

'What do you mean?' I shout over the music, following his gaze to the few guys our own age.

'They're like eighteen maybe … they're young,' he tells me, with a shrug.

'Oh,' I say, my mind jolting with the realisation they're not my age.

I sip my drink. One breath. One step. One breath. One step. I look again at the men who are our age and for which I feel far too young for. I don't belong to this world. Stop it, I order myself. Fake it until you feel it. I smile at Logan, Stephen and some other girl, who keeps trying it on with Stephen … much to Logan and Cass's drunken amusement. We dance away together as Jessica starts dancing with some guy.

'Joy, he's been trying to catch your eye for ages,' Jessica says in my ear, coming up behind me and making me jump.

I look around to see a man watching me shyly. I smile. Everything seems funny if I make it so and I can't hide how nice it is to have something to smile about.

'Oh crap,' I laugh, as he comes over.

Jessica laughs and shoves me forwards.

'Hi, how are you?' He has to stoop a little so I can hear him over the music.

'I'm good. You?'

'I'm good. Is one of them your boyfriend?' he asks, looking at Stephen and Logan, who are watching from behind me.

I laugh. 'No.'

'Good,' he says, holding out his hand for me to take.

I look at it and then at him and think … what the heck.

He tries to lead me further into the dancefloor and away from my group of people but I hold fast – I'm not leaving them for anything.

He smiles, nods and then holds up his free arm in surrender. We dance and dance, our bodies getting closer and closer. I'm aware of his head close to my neck, of knowing instinctually that he wants to kiss me but I don't let him until I decide I might as well. I lean back a little and look at him. His eyes are lined slightly as people our age apparently are. I don't find it attractive, but I guess I'll have to learn to; then I lean in to let him kiss me. I wasn't sure I'd remember how but unlike leaving the house, this isn't something I forgot. I gently place my hand on his cheek, his slightly stubbled chin rubbing sharply against my face, making me want to recoil for the unfamiliarity of it.

I pull away after a moment, acutely aware of all the people around us. I glance about self-consciously to see if anyone was watching, only to find my group of people staring at me in surprise.

'Go Joy!' yells Jessica.

I cringe but a part of me doesn't care.

'Another drink?' Logan asks.

'Yes,' I agree enthusiastically.

'I'll catch you before the place shuts?' the guy I kissed asks me.

'Thanks, but don't worry about it,' I state.

'Oh, ok,' he says, looking slightly baffled and a little disappointed.

'Sugar coat it for him, why don't you,' Logan roars with mirth, putting his arm around me as we head off the dancefloor.

Ten minutes later, the music abruptly stops mid-song and it's announced the New Year is approaching. Logan and I race, along with everyone else, to find our friends. With our group reformed, we hold hands just in time to count down to the New Year in FIVE, FOUR, THREE, TWO, ONE ... HAPPY NEW YEAR!

And for once ... I think it is.

Chapter Twenty

JOYCE – AGE 24

I moved into my bedroom a few days after New Year. For the first time, my life felt too big for the narrow existence held within that sofa bed. Like a hermit crab who's outgrown their shell, I needed to find a new one.

It feels good to be reunited with the snow-covered mountains outside my window. As I lie in my bed, the shadow of a smile crosses my face as I recall coming home at 5.40am on New Year's Day and laughing the entire way. Aunt Beth had left me a hot water bottle in my bed, which I was eternally grateful for because I was chilled and in agony to my core – I ran on pure elation that night and I adored it. I remember sneaking upstairs and whispering into Aunt Beth's darkened room that I was home and her grunt of acknowledgement. I took a plate of gluten-free toast and a hot chocolate, which has no added sugar, to my sofa bed, and watched TV as I munched – the irony of having a sugar-free beverage when I'd just drunk half a bar made me giggle. I went to bed exhausted, my body hating me for making it stand and dance and just generally function but I fell asleep smiling because, for once, what was good outstripped what was bad. The warmth inside me from being around people didn't fade away like I'm used to it doing, it didn't become bittersweet or painful … it remained, glowing gloriously inside me.

I stretch, my joints popping, my head groggy from sleep. I roll over and pick up my phone before getting up for the day, my eyes squinting against the bright screen.

Logan: Get ready … we're going to Maltdonia!

Logan: The host of the hostel you really liked wants us to go!

Logan: Get packing … we're going travelling!

Logan again: I'm coming home this weekend so we can book flights and arrange everything we need.

Logan: Sorry forgot to say I messaged them.

Logan: Get packing!

I stare at the screen, confused and utterly uncomprehending.

'Ohhhh,' I sound out loud, as the drunken memory strikes me. 'The TravelerStay.'

I struggle to sit upright, a concoction of bubbling, squirming and churning emotions brewing inside me but as I catch sight of myself in the mirror, eyes heavy with bags, skin pale and drawn, my limbs still weak from yesterday's activities. All sensation fades as my reality sinks in.

Over the next few days, I wait for Logan with growing doubt. It comes in layers like the snow outside – each day I awaken to a fresh dusting of hope which thaws into reality. I feel like I have emotional whiplash from the extremes of hope and dread. Everything's happening so fast and I can't seem to grab a hold of it, but I know I don't want it to stop because the further I go, the further away I am from the person I was.

Dog watches me as I pace the kitchen, putting away odd bits and bobs … trying to pass the time until Logan arrives. He turns up on my doorstep, bang on twelve o'clock, as we'd arranged. When I open the door, he sweeps me up into a huge hug.

'We're going to Maltdonia!' he cries excitedly, lifting me up off my feet and spinning me around.

'Haha, stop you'll make me dizzy!' I yell, clinging onto him.

Dog grumbles from the end of the hall – clearly unsure if he should be joining the excitement or protecting me.

'Right, first things first. We need to check your passport's in date. Then we need to get travel insurance – I'm guessing you don't have any – and then we can book our flights.'

'Wait, when are they wanting us to come?'

'Two weeks from now.'

'That soon,' I say, taken aback.

'Nah, that's plenty of time.'

'What about your uni?' I ask, looking for an out.

'Joy, I graduated last summer,' he says with an amused look. 'You got me a hipflask with an engraving of my name, the date of my graduation and my uni motto on it.'

'I did?' I say uncertainly.

'You did.'

'That's a thoughtful gift,' I say, surprised by myself.

'It was,' he laughs. 'Come on.'

I follow Logan to the kitchen, where my laptop is already set up for us to use.

'Logan, are you sure this is a good idea? I can't work, I can't …' my words trail away as my eyes partake in a detailed examination of the tiles on the floor.

'Yeah, but I'm with you. I'll help with everything. If you're tired one night then I can cover your shift. It's only a few nights you work and you can sleep during the shift – plus you get two days off a week. Even if you spend the rest of that time in bed at least you're doing it somewhere different,' he says earnestly. 'If it doesn't work out you can always come home. It's not like you're tied into staying, it's voluntary you being there.'

'Ok ...' I say meekly. 'Let's just see how much all of this is going to cost first.'

Trying to find insurance was a nightmare, mostly because none of the insurance companies had heard of Lyme disease and didn't have it as a pre-existing condition to choose from. In the end we had to call them up to get them to create a whole new code to enter into the website. Two exhausting and frustrating hours later, we get there. Then come the flights. I was expecting them to be a huge cost but surprisingly they weren't. I insist on getting wheelchair assistance even though Logan doesn't think I need it. I watch him as he clicks away on my laptop, arranging everything, unsure if he's overestimating my abilities or if I'm underestimating them. As we get closer to confirming our bookings, my fingers dig deeper into the sides of my thighs.

'You ready?' Logan asks keenly, hovering over the button to confirm our booking.

'No, wait ...' I fluster.

'Look, why don't we book them and if you really don't want to come then there's a 24-hour cancellation. So, you can cancel your ticket.'

'Will you still go if I don't?'

'Yeah, I can't wait,' he says, as though the answer was obvious.

I can feel my face cringing as I watch the subtle pressure on his finger increase until it goes click. The screen goes blank and then the page reloads with the message: Your booking is confirmed!

'Now all you have to do,' Logan says with trepidation, 'is tell Aunt Beth.'

It's strange, to sit before someone with information you know they won't like but which you have to tell them. The TV is on but I can't focus on it. I keep snatching glances at Aunt Beth, debating when and how to tell her, but after my sixth glance at her she takes the debate out of my control.

'What's wrong?' Aunt Beth asks, catching me looking at her

'Nothing,' I say a little too quickly. 'Actually, you know how Logan goes travelling a lot, well, he's been given the opportunity to go to Maltdonia to work in exchange for his accommodation and food.'

'That boy travels everywhere,' she mutters. 'That's good news though, shame if it means he won't be about, but good for him. Is this part of his year off between uni and starting work?'

I sit up a little straighter, encouraged.

'I think so … he's asked me if I'll come with him,' I say, the words sticking slightly in my throat.

Aunt Beth freezes. I watch her apprehensively; I'm not entirely convinced she's still breathing. Slowly, like ice thawing, she comes back to life.

'And … eh … what – what did you say?'

'I-I said yes—' I blanch at the brittle look on her face and quickly add, 'that I'll think about it. It's an amazing opportunity and he's asked me to come along. We only work a couple of hours each day and the rest of the time is ours to do what we want with.' Even to me, my voice sounds desperate.

We sit in silence, Aunt Beth still staring determinedly at the TV. I sigh, give up and join her in looking at the TV without actually watching it. After a moment, she turns the volume down and looks to me, her face unreadable.

'Where will you be working? And what kind of work will you be doing?'

'In a hostel,' I answer. 'So, cleaning, chatting to guests, checking them in and out … that kind of stuff.'

'And where will you sleep?'

'In a dormitory with other workers,' I explain.

I sit still, frozen in place as though any movement I make might sway her.

'You've not thought this through, Joyce. How do you know that they won't rope you in to do more work than you've agreed to do? You struggle enough with sleep here so how are you going to cope sharing a room with a group of strangers? Hostels are loud and busy places, you'll constantly be around people with no privacy, no peace, no downtime – how are you going to manage that? What's more, everything will be different, the currency will be different, the culture will be different, the language, the food. How will you cope in the heat? Will you be able to maintain your diet there? What happens if you get sick and need someone to look after you. What …'

Her words keep coming but they've become blurred, hazy, incomprehensible noise to me now. I look at the picture of the four of us on the mantelpiece, as I feel myself shrinking. I hadn't noticed how much I'd grown until she'd punctured me. Each word she utters compresses me until I feel so small, so hopeless and so broken that I feel like I'm nothing.

'Fine, I'll tell him no,' I say, cutting her off and leaving the room.

Chapter Twenty-one

LOGAN – AGE 25

The best things you can say/send to a sick person or their caregiver
- You look great but how do you actually feel?
- We'll plan to meet up but if you're not able to then no worries.
- I'm not going to lie; I've no idea what to say but I'm here for you.
- Can I help with anything while I'm here?
- I know how hard you're trying.
- I believe you.

A personal favourite
- No need to reply, just wanted you to know I was thinking of you!

I smirk a little as I look at the screen of my phone. I was waiting for this message.

Joy: Hey, can we meet up? Maybe go for a walk at the woods?

Me: Sure thing. Meet in an hour? Want a lift?

Three minutes later.

Joy: Thanks, but AB is passing there anyway.

A good hour later, I park up on the edge of the nearby estate. I wait ten minutes before messaging Joy to ask where she is.

Joy: I'm at the gates, where are you?

Me: Haha, I parked at the other end.

Joy: Meet in the middle?

Me: See you in a bit.

I head into the estate, carefully picking out the least icy route. I head over the stone bridge, keeping my arms out to steady myself on the ice. Half way, I pause to lean over the edge of the bridge to see the heavy gush of water beneath me, my toes near its rim, I'm amazed no cars have gone over it given it has no sides. Once I cross the bridge, I walk along the edge of the icy road rather than on it, my trainers making a squeaky crunch as they sink into the snow piled up on its edges. The red streaks on my trainers standing out starkly against the bright white of the snow.

'Hi,' I call ten minutes later as the oversized figure of Joy comes into view, I can't resist a smile at the mass of thermals she has on.

'Hey,' she calls back, sounding a little out of breath.

I hold out my arms to give her a hug once she's in reaching distance, her many layers making her as soft and sinkable as a marshmallow.

'So ... what's Beth said to put you off,' I say with amusement, my breath coming out in a white mist.

'How did you know?' she asks, frowning a little.

'Because I know her and I know you.' I say, fidgeting with my watch strap; it's been fighting with my sleeve since this morning. 'Have you got any zips amongst those layers?'

'Yeah,' she says, pulling her hands out of her pockets to show me.

'Can I give you this?' I ask, taking my watch off and handing it to her.

She shoves it in her pocket and zips it up. We slowly wander down a thin side path, off the main estate road and into the woods, the branches above our heads sagging with snow as though they're tired of the effort of holding themselves up.

'So, what's she saying?' I ask, kicking at the snow with my toe while we walk.

'She just pointed some things out … She basically said that I wouldn't be able to cope with working and with how busy hostels can be.'

'Ok,' I say slowly, thinking through my response. 'You know at this time of year it'll be low season so it shouldn't be busy. That's why I thought going now was a good idea.'

'Yeah but everything will be different, the food, money, people …' Joy says, ducking to go under a low-hanging branch.

I resist the urge to shake it as she stoops.

'That's the whole point,' I laugh. 'Things aren't meant to be the same. That's the adventure in discovering all these different places and things. And they have supermarkets! You'll be able to get things that you can eat.'

'What if I end up needing to go to the doctors?' she frets.

'Joy, they have hospitals.'

'I know, but Aunt Beth doesn't think—'

'Joy, you're an adult. You don't need Beth's permission or her approval. You have to do what's best for you. Look …' I say, coming to a stop so I can face her. I open my mouth but pause. What if she's not well enough? Who am I to know? 'We can cancel if you really don't want to go but I really want you there and I don't want you to not go because you're worried about something happening which might never happen. You've fought so hard to get better; do you really want to spend your life being stuck here?'

'I'm still ill,' she says bleakly, staring off into the trees.

'I know, but you'll always be ill, Joy. I've watched you get sicker and better and sicker and then better again but your life is more than just that and you should get to spend the better bits doing things that are fun and exciting. If anyone's earned it, you have. This disease can't be your life, Joy.'

She looks at me then, just for a moment, before looking away again. I feel like I've struck a match – I'm just not sure if it'll burn into fruition or futility.

'I don't know,' she finally says.

'I just, I honestly think this will be the making of you. So, are you in or are you out?'

'… I'm in,' she says hesitantly.

'Promise?' I say, not entirely feigning my dubiousness.

'Yes,' she says, a smile beginning to brighten her eyes.

'You promise, no matter what happens, you'll go?'

'Yes,' she says, with a note of laughter. 'I promise I'll go … no matter what!'

'I'm holding you to that,' I insist. 'I better head home, do you want a lift?'

'Thanks, but I want to walk a bit – plus Aunt Beth said she'd pick me up on her way home.'

'Ok, well, be careful, it's really slippery,' I remind her, huddling my shoulders together against the cold. 'Here, the next time we see each other, we'll be flying to Maltdonia!'

'Promise!' she laughs.

'Promise,' I call back, as I turn to leave.

A lightness in my step and a grin on my face.

Chapter Twenty-two

JOYCE – AGE 24

It feels strange to walk alone without a soul in sight; it leaves an odd sense of vulnerability, of being exposed, but it's also freeing having only myself to tend to. I dig my icy hands into my pockets, my fingers finding something unknown. When I pull the object out, I find Logan's watch in my hand. I automatically turn around as though expecting to find him racing after me to retrieve it but, of course, he's not.

I hurry back the way I came, slipping and sliding on the treacherous path, taking every shortcut I know. I keep to the snowy verge which runs along the main road of the estate, the towering trees and the river to the left of me, a verge of trees and fields beyond them to the right. I shiver as I remove my glove so that I can call him but there's no answer. He's possibly driving if he's reached his car already, I consider but as I near the bridge Logan's car slowly comes into view through the bare trees.

'Logan,' I call, looking around me as though hoping he'll hop out from behind the trees.

'Logan!'

I try calling him again, the silence between hitting the green button and the first ring seems to take an eternity. Buuup my phone sounds in my ear and at the exact same time comes a

Brrrr-ing noise. I slowly lower my phone so I can hear the Brrr-ing more clearly. I look around, trying to discern where the noise is coming from. I move my head this way and that, growing increasingly frustrated because my old hearing would have detected the direction immediately. When the phone goes quiet, I call it again, wandering a little down the road towards the bridge. I pause as I catch sight of a black blot standing starkly against the white snowy edging of the bridge. I shake my head a little – this is how Logan goes through more phones than I do pills. I head towards it, my first step on the bridge sending my legs splaying but, somehow, I steady myself, my hand reaching for my racing heart. This time I take a more cautious step. I stoop to pick up the ringing phone, which is flashing my name on its screen.

'Logan,' I yell, staring about me, an uneasy sense seizing my soul. 'Logan!'

My eyes sweep over the ground near the phone, the confusion of footprints in the snow lining the edge of the bridge coming to a startling stop, the snow around it becomes compact, compressed, scattered and missing. I lean over the edge, a streak of bright red staring up at me through the depth of the dark water.

'Logan,' I whisper breathlessly, my heart lurching.

I slither and slide across the ice to reach the other side. As soon as I hit the snowy verge, I run. My feet slipping as I slide down the embankment, my hands out before me to steady my descent. I plunge straight into the water, its icy depths seizing my legs in its vice as I wade out to hip height. The current's not strong but it's strong enough to push me and hold me back as though trying to spare me from the sight before me.

I forge forwards, relief pulsing through me as I reach him. I grab his arms and roll him over so his face isn't under the water but as soon as I lift him off the rocks, which partly hold him, the river pulls at him to take him away from me. I grab him under each arm and drag him backwards towards the embankment. I'm almost at the edge when my feet slip and slide out from beneath me, Logan's lifeless body tipping me over, his face the grey pallor of death, which I know too well. My breath comes in stuttering gasps as my ribs and hip smash onto the rocks. For a moment I forget how to breathe, my eyes locking onto a bloodless wound gaping at me on the back of his skull. I try not to look at it as I struggle onto my feet and stumble my way out of the water, pulling and dragging Logan with me until we're free of the waters grasp.

I know, even before I check his pulse, that his life is gone but hope defies me. I check again, his neck, his wrist … but there's nothing but stillness. I frantically feel in my pockets for my phone but it's not there. I tip back Logan's head to check his airways before pinching his nose and covering his mouth with mine. I breathe into him until I see his chest swell and then hasten to start chest compressions.

'Help!' I scream breathlessly, my voice so desperate it scares me. 'Help!'

I push down hard on his chest, over and over again, his ribs compressing and pushing back against my hands. I feel my body floundering, I see it in the weakening effects my efforts have on his chest. I gaps for air, my heart hammering, unsure if I should stop to find my phone and call for help or keep going.

'Someone, please,' I shout, but only the river replies.

'HELP!' I've never felt so alone.

I push down hard on his chest, using all the force I have.

'HE—' I try to cry but there isn't enough air in my chest.

'Hey,' a voice shouts.

I look up to see a man, a woman and their dog hurrying down the slope towards me.

'Call an ambulance,' I gasp.

The man stops to pull out his phone while the woman continues towards me, the dog stopped halfway between its owners – wary of approaching.

'How long's he been in the water?' she asks.

'I don't know,' I say breathlessly, my back, arms, legs … everything burning with the cold and the heat of exhaustion.

'You're doing great but let me take over,' she says gently.

'No,' I say, even though I know I can't keep going, I push down harder.

'You're getting tired, let me take over.'

'No.'

'I know what I'm doing. Trust me,' she says. 'On the count of three. One. Two. Three.'

I throw myself backwards into the snow and she immediately takes my place. I watch her as I sit in the purity of the snow, the cold air stinging my eyes, which stare wide and unblinking. I feel the horror being carved on my face at the sound of Logan's ribs beginning to break under the repeated force upon them.

I don't know how long it takes for the ambulance to arrive, for them to take over, to put him on a stretcher and load him into the ambulance. I find a blanket around my shoulders … I don't know how it got there. Two phones are pressed into my hand as I pass the man who's still standing at the top of the slope. I'm led into the ambulance and sat down. Sirens scream like the call of death. I close my eyes as Logan's body is worked on. Unable to bear seeing him broken any further, I barely feel the movement as we hurtle towards the hospital. We all know he's dead. It's just that no one is allowed to say it yet and until they do … I cling to hope.

Logan is taken away from me in such a rush that I can't protest. I'm ushered into a cubicle and checked over before being led into a waiting room in a daze. I'm given some dry scrubs to put on by a kind nurse who saw me shivering. I sit alone and I vaguely wonder why. Two police officers come in and pull up two chairs in front of me. They ask me questions. I answer although my voice doesn't sound like mine anymore. I expect them to be harsh, to try to contradict me like they do on TV but they're kind, gentle even. One of them puts a hand on my shoulder at one point and I'm confused as to why but then I notice the droplets on my scrubs … I must be crying. They offer to call Aunt Beth. I thank them and give them Logan's phone. They leave me.

I look up in time to see, through the glass window in the door, Logan's mum and dad being ushered into the waiting room opposite mine. They sit down and the doctor with them does the same. I stand up so I can watch in the silence as their lips move, as they freeze in the moment between impending doom and it hitting them. I wish I hadn't, but I make myself watch as their lives are changed irrevocably. As Logan's dad slumps forward, his head in his hands as he weeps and as Logan's mum wraps her arms around him, their heads buried together. I stumble a step backwards as though shoved by the impact of what I've seen, my legs hitting the rim of the chair with such force that I fall back into the seat, numb to my pain.

Chapter Twenty-three

JOYCE – AGE 25

The cruellest realities:

1) You think you're safe, that the caged world you live in is all there is and everything beyond it hasn't changed since you left it but that's an illusion forged as a means to cope. Outside, life goes on, catastrophes occur, pain ensues and just because we're sick … it doesn't stop the forces from outside coming crashing in.

2) I'd like to think being chronically sick is enough to deal with but life doesn't give you a reprieve. You'll get sick on top of being sick, your organs will get damaged from treatment, you'll end up developing some other disease because the one you already have makes you susceptible, you'll lose your home, you'll lose your loved ones, you'll lose whatever you hold dear because the world doesn't care if you've already gone through enough – it doesn't care that you're already on the edge of breaking.

3) You can do everything right, absolutely everything and still … it will never be enough.

It was ruled an accident and his body was released a week later. He died from a head wound from where he fell on the ice. It was a freak accident in the way that his head hit the ground; the chances were tiny but he always had a way of beating the odds. They said his lifeless body had no means of stopping itself as he slipped over the side of the bridge. They found no water in his lungs, he died before he hit it. Small mercies.

I stare at myself in the mirror. I look like a ghost. I'm dressed in a fitted black dress, black shoes ... his mum and dad are traditionalists. Stephen set up a group chat of the old school group and said that we should wear something bright underneath or in our pockets. I suggested underwear – everyone agreed. So now, under my sombre attire, are the brightest most multicoloured pants and bra that I could find. The bra doesn't fit. It doesn't matter. The pain the wire inflicts is a reminder that it's there.

Logan's mum and dad arranged for a funeral car to pick us all up. When I clamber into it, it's already full. I sit next to Stephen, it's the only seat left. The car contains the old gang ... a reunion none expected. We greet each other with hushed hellos, nods of acknowledgement, the occasional faint smile of solidarity. Some of the them have their arms around each other, some openly cry. I simply sit.

I follow as we step out of the car and head into the church, greeting each member of Logan's family as we pass them on the way in. Davey, Logan's uncle, gives me a hug and a tight-lipped nod. Logan's dad shakes my hand but he doesn't meet my eye. His mum hugs me and asks if I'll join Stephen in the front row – I don't see how I can refuse.

I lower myself onto the cushioned bench, the hard-wooden back of the pew already making mine ache. Stephen and I look at each other, a moment of unspoken reconciliation passing between us for this day. I look into his eyes, they're so etched with pain that it's easy to forget all the anguish he placed in mine. I hold my hand out to him and I'm glad when he takes it. As the service starts, we both look ahead, staring at the coffin encasing our best friend.

The service feels like it will never end and yet when it does it comes as a surprise. We all stand as the body is carried outside, we follow numbly after him. Outside, the freshness of winter whispers about us. We walk the short way down the country road to the graveyard. Our steps summoned by the piper's lament. Once again, Stephen and I are near the front, walking behind Logan's family – his body leading the way in the warmth of the hearse. It seems cruel to me, to take him from the warmth only to put him in the cold. We mill about on the short grass and the on the thin path near Logan's new home, waiting for the minister to start speaking. A few people I knew from school come up to me, overwrought with grief and seeking comfort in mutual sorrow. I'm hugging Cass when I catch Stephen looking about. I let Cass go, instantly I know it's me he seeks. I gently push to the front of the crowd until I'm at the front beside him. I watch while Logan's mum and dad step up, on either side of Logan's grave. They're each handed a length of gold rope for lowering him down. Two of his brothers come next, with Stephen and me at the end. We were asked before the funeral if we would help lower him. I said yes even though I was worried I'd drop him. I almost smile as I imagine his dead body coming to life to roar with mirth at my mistake but the lowering is all for show … it's done mechanically. I'm handed the gold silk rope and told to hold it just so and to let it slide through my hand.

Logan's coffin is slowly lowered into the ground, taken from the glow of winter sun into the darkness. I dread the moment we have to drop the cord and let go of him. Stephen and I are the last pair to drop ours. I can't help but inwardly feel the dull thud of the heavy gold rope hitting him. The minister reads from a sheet of paper. There's only one part of it I hear, though. The words, so clearly from his family, are jarring coming from the minister's mouth.

'We will never see you again in this world but we will hold you all the tighter in the next.'

I look at the crowd around me as we walk, Logan's friends and I with our secretly vibrant underwear hidden in an ocean of black, all moving back along to the road towards the hotel for refreshments. I never understood why people wore black to funerals, the deepest of colours, but I understand now … we are the shadows of death. We walk in a procession of the mourning but the mourning don't cry for the body that's been buried; they cry for themselves, they cry for their loss, the regret, the things left unsaid, the grief and finality of another's departure.

When we get to the hotel, the old gang congregate together in the function room where food and drink are being served. We order Logan's favourite, a whisky whose name I instantly forget but whose price is heavy enough to make Logan proud of us for trying it. The heat it spreads from the back of my throat to the pit of my stomach is comforting. We chat, share stories, vow to go for a night out in memory of our friend. They talk of the time Logan saw someone drop their wallet, picked it up and returned it to them, only to find he'd returned it to the person who'd stolen it. In turn, I tell them about the condom bombs and the shed. It's strange, the conversations are mundane, everyday topics and yet it feels abnormal. When no one is looking, we flash a little of what we're wearing to show that we've worn something bright. Laughing at Stephen's luminous green boxers, I glance towards Logan's family to see if they heard us and disapprove but only his mum seems to have heard and is watching us with a sad smile.

When the car comes to pick us up to take us all home, we go over as a group to say goodbye to Logan's family.

'You look after yourself won't you,' Davey tells me, his voice drowning with emotion, 'and remember you were Logan's friend so you're a friend to us too.'

'I will, so long as you do the same,' I say, hugging him once more.

When I get to Logan's dad, I open my mouth but nothing comes out. We simply look at each other, pain and loss passing between us so distinctly that no words are needed. I put my hand in my jacket pocket, my fingers closing tightly around Logan's watch. I know I need to return it but as I reach his mum and, she pulls me into a hug, my hand leaves my pocket empty.

'You did everything you could,' she whispers into my ear, sending a chill down my spine.

She pulls away from me but doesn't let go of my arms. I nod, looking into her piercing eyes which mirror Logan's. She squeezes my arms and lets me go. I walk numbly towards the door where those who've said goodbye are already waiting. I glance back. I can't do it. I can't give back the only thing I have left of him.

Chapter Twenty-four

JOYCE – AGE 25

I sit in my window seat, looking out to the mountains still covered in snow and ice but its beauty has lost its innocence now. Logan and I had said that we'd try and climb them in the summer. I hold his watch in my hand. Time passes.

I keep busy. I do all the things I did before he died but they're far harder than they were before. My body tires quicker, my brain doesn't focus, my heart doesn't want to beat. I try to smile but the act I'd perfected to the world no longer comes with ease. It's an effort and I no longer care to enact it. Fake it until you feel it … I thought if I displayed it outwardly, I'd eventually feel it inwardly but it was superficial, surface deep – I see that now. Still, it was better than living like this.

Late that afternoon, I log into my emails to check if anything's been sent about my course. There's one email which catches my eye though – an email notification from TravelerStay.

Host message:

From all of us at Ohana Hostel,

We are deeply saddened to hear that Logan has passed away. Although we never met him, just by the messages we exchanged, we could tell what a remarkable man he was. We completely understand if you would like to cancel your TravelerStay with us but should you wish to come – we'd be very happy to welcome you into our family with warm and open arms.

If you could please let us know your plans, at your earliest convenience, we'd be very grateful.

The Ohana team

I stare at the message, unable to take it in fully until I read it again. I rest my head in my hands for a moment. I'd forgotten all about it. With a sigh, I click out of the email and look at the one under it. Boarding pass it reads at the top; followed by instructions to print them off. I lean back in my chair at the kitchen table, my mind blank. I rub at the heavy weight on my chest, as though rubbing it in will make it go away, before picking up my phone and unlocking it, my finger hovering over the icon to go into my messages – but I can't bring myself to open it. I know there's one in there from Logan, unopened and unread but I can't open it knowing that I'll never get another message from him again.

'You promise, no matter what happens, you'll go?' his voice whispers in my ear.

'Yes,' my own voice rings with laughter. *'I promise I'll go … no matter what!'*

I shake my head. How can you hold me to that now? I slam the lid of my laptop shut and stare numbly out to the darkening world outside the kitchen window. Odd flecks of snow mixed with heavy rain hit the window. I slowly get to my feet and walk to the back door. Opening it, I step outside into the darkness and sit on the bench before the shed, the icy sting of the dregs of winter lashing my skin.

I wrap my arms around my ribs but I feel like they might sink straight through me; it's as though I'm not really here at all. I release one hand and use it to grip onto the wet arm of the bench, squeezing it tightly until my fingers go pale, just to feel something of substance. I look at my thighs as the rain and sleet infiltrate my jeans and a coolness seeps across my flesh.

No tears fall from my eyes but something somewhere inside me is breaking, being beaten. I can feel its pain but it's like it doesn't belong to me. I feel like the shadow of all that I was becoming, is now dying. My body shivers but I barely feel the coldness biting into me. I don't know how to stop the nothingness from encasing me.

I get to my feet and move closer to the shed with a sense of controlled elegance that I don't feel. I study the shed. The colours bright but less vibrant with the weathering of time. I stand before it, running my hand over the lumps and bumps where the paint ran like tears. Slowly I crouch beside the left-hand corner, letting my fingers trace where Logan carved our names and the date of our deformation.

I place my hand over it and hold it there as though, somehow, I'll be holding him too. I feel something warm and wet nudging my outstretched arm. When I look up, I find myself staring into Dog's sorrowful eyes and I instantly wrap my arms around him.

'Don't ever leave me,' I whisper into his rain-soaked coat.

I don't know how long we sit there in the drizzling rain and sleet but slowly I pull away from him. I numbly remove my phone from my pocket and open Logan's message.

Logan: I, Joy Jack, have promised to go to Maltdonia no matter what. No backing out now, it's in writing … kind of. See you at the check-in.

I clutch my phone, looking up at the stars which wink away at me through gaps in the cloud, as though they're in on it. I close my eyes as I listen to his voice hidden in the breeze, *'I honestly think this will be the making of you.'*

I replay his words over and over again. I don't ever want to forget the sound of his voice. I'm not scared of going anymore. I'm not scared of anything. That's the freedom of indifference. So, why not go? His voice whispers to me. With numb fingers, I use my phone to print the boarding pass – wiping at the screen smeared with droplets. I slowly get up with stiff but determined legs. I need to pack.

'You having a clear out?' Aunt Beth asks an hour later, leaning against the doorway of my room, to check on me after finishing work.

'No, I'm going to Maltdonia,' I tell her, distractedly.

I examine two pairs of jeans. I don't know what I need to take and what I don't. Pack light, I order myself, dumping the second pair for leggings instead.

'Joyce … Joyce, you can't,' she says, sounding stunned.

'Why?' I ask, comparing a hoodie verses a jumper … I pick the hoodie.

'Because Logan's …' she stops.

'Dead,' I supply. 'He's dead but I'm not and I promised him. I promised I'd go.'

'I appreciate you want to honour your friend,' she says, her words painfully measured, her body now rigidly upright, 'but Logan wouldn't expect you to go without him and if it was going be to a challenge to do this with him then how will you manage alone?'

'No idea,' I say flippantly.

'Joyce—'

'I'm not Joyce!' I exclaim. 'Joyce is gone. I'm not her anymore and I need you to let me do this.'

Aunt Beth looks crestfallen. She lowers her head for a moment and then turns and shuts the door meekly behind her. I sink onto my bed, riddled with guilt.

Chapter Twenty-five

JOY – AGE 25

Is this cheating? It certainly feels like it. Only I feel no danger, no thrill from the risk of exposure. Isn't there meant to be some reward for jeopardising your morality? Or is this feeling of enforced submission my reprimand for taking something I have no right to claim? I seem to have done that a lot recently, I think, looking at Logan's watch on my thin wrist. Its face is forever looking downward. It's like it's hiding from me, trying to delay the moment we come face to face – ashamed. In reality, the straps are too large and my fear of defiling it prevents me from creating a new hole for the metal tooth to pierce.

I roll down the tarmac in an ancient wheelchair, the repetitive but intermittent elevation on the right-hand side, from whatever is stuck on the wheel, making me feel like a wonky trolley that might rebel in any direction. I could have walked but instead I cheated and ticked the box which said I needed the wheelchair. I don't know if I should hold my head down or hold my head high. This isn't a role I'm prepared for. I'm not prepared for any of this.

'Ready?' the man behind my chair asks.

I stare up at the vast machine before me. Its size astounds me, yet the flapless wings of this mighty bird will take me somewhere far from everything I've ever known. I get slowly to my feet, one hand still on the arm of the wheelchair for balance. I gaze at the metal stairs leading into the neck of the plane before turning to look at the man who, for the last thirty minutes, has had control over my every move.

'Thank you,' I say automatically, reaching for my carry-on.

'I'll take it,' the guy offers, pulling my small case from under the seat of the wheelchair – the perfect helper.

I thank him again as I reach a hand for the rail of the stairs. Taking my first step tentatively, testing my strength. I feel the eyes of my fellow disabled and their handlers below me and the eyes of the crew above me ... watching, assessing, wondering just how sick or injured I am. The fascination is all the stronger for the oddity of me being young. I've used the wheelchair assistance for a reason they cannot see but their watchful examination puts me under pressure to conform to the expectations of the roll they want to cast me into. Unfortunately for them, my reclaimed strength renders that outward visibility of disability they seek unrewarded. I'm stiff and aching, granted, from sitting in that prison chair for the last three hours but my legs hold me strong as I make my way up the steps of the plane.

I pause as I enter the plane and as my boarding pass is taken from me before I'm led to my seat. My case is placed in the locker above my head and once again I thank the man for his kindness. We, the sick, habitually waver between being forever grateful and forever bitter – most frequently we're both. Our bodies constantly shredded from the double-edged sword we're struck with in exchange for functionality. I sink into my seat before watching the line of people being led, from inside the airport, out to the plane like sheep being herded through a gate and I'm relieved that I got to board before them. While people find their seats, I squirm in mine, trying to find a position that isn't uncomfortable; I fail. I keep telling myself that in four hours I won't have to play into anyone's role other than my own. I can do this, I tell myself, my breathing growing heavy. I can do this.

'Thank you for joining our flight today to the Island of Maltdonia …' The captain's breathy voice crackles into the now still cabin.

Have they already locked the doors? I strain to see over the rows of chairs in front of me. They must have because everyone's seated and the safety demonstrations are underway. There's no going back; there can be no return. The smooth fabric of my leggings is soft and supple under the vice grasp of my hands. You can still go home as soon as you land, I remind myself, you don't even have to leave the airport. I order myself to loosen my grip. I made my choice … I will not be afraid of it. Besides, what's the alternative?

Outside my window, the world is moving slowly. I know I should be paying attention to the demonstration but I can't help but watch as the plane turns on the runway. We spin like a slow-motion ballet dancer – seemingly moving from one point of contact with the ground. The plane pauses before we thunder forwards; my body pushed backwards by the vice grip of the plane's momentum. I rest my head back, releasing the tension of the pressure from the plane's force. Around me, some grip their armrests, others close their eyes, some don't even seem to notice as the wheels leave the ground … I smile because as we enter the air and the oxygen outside declines I feel, for the first time, that I can breathe.

Chapter Twenty-six

JOY – AGE 25

This is why I cheated, I think to myself as I exit the plane and the only wheelchair available is taken by someone in greater need than myself.

I walk, with somewhat brittle legs, down the corridor of the airport – my small suitcase rolling behind me like an old faithful companion. The force of my movement and my relief at arriving in a functioning body slowly expelling my residual stiffness. I head straight through baggage collection, where groups of people huddle around the conveyer belt waiting for the black-tongued serpent to expel their luggage from its gaping mouth.

The curving corridor, whose walls are papered with posters of various attractions, opens up into the bowels of the airport where lines of people wait to check in and where others peruse the gift shops. I grip tightly onto the handle of Old Faithful as I allow the stream of people off my flight to lead me outside.

As I walk through the automatic doors, the warm air from outside blasts against my skin. The bright sun blinding me as the air is momentarily snatched from my lungs before the country's warm breathless air, acidic with the smell of petrol and other fumes, re-enters my clean country lungs. I rummage frantically inside my bag for my sunglasses, then take a breath as I stare around me, my sensitive eyes struggling to grow accustomed to the brightness. To the right I spot a bus towards the end of the building with a line of people slowly boarding it. Tentatively, I head over to the lady who's standing near the back dishing out tickets.

'Where to?' she asks, barely looking at me.

'The city centre,' I tell her.

She prints me a ticket and I exchange it for 200 Maltdonian Nix.

I'm the last to get on and so I have no choice but to take the only seat available. I try a friendly smile at the girl I'm forced to sit next to but the girl looks sourly unimpressed by my arrival.

Within minutes of being on the bus, buds of sweat bloom on my back as my insides bubble and boil with the heat. I tie my hair up so that it's off my neck but the relief it creates is fleeting. I feel like I'm being pushed into my seat as the heaviness settles into my body – a warning sign that worse might come. I try to distract myself from the knot that's tying in my intestines by studying the mountainous terrain we're driving through. I don't know why, maybe because I knew how warm the summers are here, but I thought the land would be less like home – less green with less vegetation, even if it is of a different variety. Slowly, I take a deep breath in before releasing it in an attempt to relax, my body growing heavier with each judder of the bus, the weight of myself setting into my bones like they're slowly being replaced with glass … heavy, dense and yet frighteningly fragile.

As we get closer to the city, the land naturally becomes more populated with houses and shops with names I can't read. The buildings grow taller and the roads grow wider.

I get off at the only stop and like everyone else I wait patiently for my turn to collect my suitcase from the luggage compartment. Slowly, I make my way to the edge of the crowd, where I'll be out the way but still within the safety of their numbers, as I try to gather myself. Glancing around me, it's reassuring that most people look as directionless as me. Like a mob of meercats, we're all straight-backed, wide-eyed, heads jerking this way and that as we search for our destinations.

'Taxi?' a man who's been lurking, like I am, at the edge of the crowd swoops in to ask me.

'No, thanks,' I say automatically, deliberately trying not to pay him much attention.

He swiftly moves on through the crowd crowing 'taxi' after every other person he passes.

I take out my phone and look at the pictures I took of the route to the hostel. My eyes hunt for any signs or street names and I find plenty, only they're not written in English like they are on my phone. My preparation in saving the route there, for which I praised myself for at the time, now seems naïve. While my skin relishes the cooling breeze, my eyes seek out landmarks instead and eventually I spot one of the many bridges that cross the river which runs through the city. Reluctantly, I turn away from the safety of the crowd and head towards it.

The river is lined on either side with stone walls, ornately carved and gleaming white just like the immaculate paths and the grand historic-looking buildings which line this side of the river. On the opposite side, there seems to be less grandeur in the buildings and more variety in cafés with outdoor seating overhung by the branches of trees. I pause at the end of the bridge, the throng quieter here. I check my phone again, my fingers fumbling with the screen, my chest tight. I have no idea where I am, I have no internet to check and limited energy to hunt for it.

On a hunch, I head left towards the sea of white walls, historic buildings and split-off pathways, Old Faithful trundling contently behind me on the smooth path, oblivious to the aching in my elbow from pulling it. My gaze slowly moves to a family ahead of me. The mother and father are walking while two girls speed ahead on their bikes before cycling back, like dogs on an extendable lead. Perhaps it's the children, but I single these parents out to be my saviours.

'Excuse me, hi, sorry. Do you know where Ohana is?' I ask before I can change my mind.

'Mhh, yes, I think it's over Eagle Bridge and then up the hill,' the lady tells me. She pauses at the uncertainty on my face before adding. 'I'll show you. Come.'

She abruptly marches onwards with me and my suitcase racing ridiculously behind her.

'Why are you here? Holiday?' the woman asks briskly, when I catch up with her.

'I'm doing a TravelerStay.' The woman scrunches her brow in confusion, so I explain, 'I'm working in exchange for my food and board.'

'And you stay here for how long?' she asks, as we continue along the riverside, her family growing further and further behind us.

'If they like me then I'll be here for a couple of months.'

'You stay here for months!' the woman says, staring at me properly for the first time. 'I hope you like it or you will not have fun.'

We pass another bridge, which seems absurdly out of place amongst the extravagance of its surrounding, its plain concrete edges crumbling and dilapidated, yet it seems to be the sole bridge dedicated to people. Eagle Bridge turns out to be as grand as it sounds; with huge statues of the great birds in flight at each corner, as though they're carrying the bridge between them.

'Go over the bridge and follow the road up the hill and, once you go up hill, then the Ohana is on the corner of third road in. Not the first, not the second but the third.'

She waves away my gratitude and wishes me luck. I mutter her instructions, over and over again as I walk over the long bridge. A constant gust of petrol fumes buffeting me with each car that goes racing past.

I'm not even partway up the hill and I'm panting like a husky in the Sahara. I pause to catch my breath at the corner of what I think is the first road that the woman was talking about. Once I've caught my breath and started to regain some feeling in my legs, I cross the road ahead of me and then cross the next until a sign on my left catches my eye which, to my greatest relief, reads Ohana Hostel.

I walk through a large stone archway in the wall, which encases the white walls and red roof of the house within it. I think of my aunt's compact cottage back home while I heave my suitcase over the well-trodden gravel drive, to a pillared folly at the front door. I don't know what I'd expected from a hostel, but it wasn't this.

'Hi, are you checking-in?' a woman's voice asks, startling me as she appears from around the side of the building, brushing at a streak of black mud on her deeply tanned leg as though she's just been gardening. I'm suddenly glad I'm in leggings – exposure to my paleness would probably blind her.

'I'm here to do the TravelerStay,' I explain.

'Ahh, you must be ...' she says brightly, inviting me to say my name but I freeze.

She tucks her long black hair behind her ear as she waits for my answer, her hooded eyes watching me with warm curiosity.

I go to answer but pause yet again. Am I Joyce or am I Joy?

'... Joy, is it?' the woman supplies, looking at me now as though questioning my IQ.

I smile. I should have known Logan would have that covered.

'Yes, sorry. It's been a long day.'

'You've had a long journey,' she excuses. 'I'm Gina. We have another girl coming soon but she hasn't actually said when she's arriving. Come in and get settled,' she adds.

It's hard to guess Gina's age; early forties maybe. Her frame looks athletic and yet you couldn't call her slim. To me she looks exotic, with beautifully rich skin. Her warm eyes are dark and with only the slightest of hairline cracks around them to hint at her age.

We enter under the folly into a room full of cubbyholes, many of which are filled with shoes.

'We ask people to take off their shoes when they enter. It helps to keep the place clean with so many people coming and going but we don't enforce it if people really don't want to. We like our volunteers to lead by example, though.'

'Right,' I say quietly.

Taking the hint, I pull off my trainers and put them in the most difficult to reach box. I follow Gina into the next room with a backward glance at the only decent pair of shoes that I have with me.

The open-plan room before me is a glowing yellow. Directly

in front of me is the kitchen area, with two corridors on either side of it, its high curving bar top separating it from the rest of the room, which is mostly monopolised by a large table and couches which line the walls. Upon them, some guests are lounging reading, listening to music and chatting quietly with one another.

It's bright and airy and the sweet scent of summer fruit and cinnamon greet me warmly. Plants climb up and along the back wall between two couches with pictures hanging from its branches of people, who I guess are past guests, like a living family tree. There's coloured string pinned to one corner of the roof and each coloured string leads to a different point in the ceiling like a shattered rainbow and there seems to be a colour chart stuck to the wall below it. It's like being in a chic nursery for grown-ups.

'Take a seat and rest. Do you want a coffee or tea?' Gina asks.

'Tea, please.'

I sit on the nearest couch, breathing deeply to try and relax my tensed limbs. There's no need to attempt to figure out who Gina is – she exudes a quiet disposition of authority simply in the way she moves.

When she reappears, she hands me a cup of tea and sits next to me on the couch.

'It was very unfortunate about your friend. I know you were meant to come together but I hope you still enjoy your time here,' Gina says gently, her head tipped to one side so her dark hair hangs out from her head like a curtain, exposing one sympathetic ear while the other's hidden from hearing.

I nod, my eyes staring down at the chipped cup in my hands, knowing I have nothing I want to say in reply.

'So, while the place is a bit quieter, you should tell me more about yourself.'

'... What would you like to know?' I ask, shuffling on the couch as though making myself comfortable rather than trying to squirm out of my own discomfort.

'Why don't you tell me about the work you do back home?'

I feel my gut knot as my insides drop. I should have been prepared for this question but my focus was dominated simply on getting here. I clasp my cup like it's my key to escape. I open my mouth and my lies begin ...

Chapter Twenty-seven

JOY – AGE 25

Once I've finished my tea, a struggle now that my nose is the size of Pinocchio's, Gina leads me past the reception desk and down a corridor to the right of the kitchen. She pauses at each of the two rooms on the right of us as we pass them. Their open doors reveal bright rooms painted peach, which are filled with metal bunkbeds with storage lockers underneath. Drawn-back curtains on each bunk reveal neatly made beds – the only blot to order being the odd suitcase or rucksack dumped at the foot of a bed.

'These are the eight- and six-bed dorms,' Gina explains.

We continue down the corridor towards a wide spiral staircase but before we reach it she gestures, with an air of the airhost's demonstration, to an open-ended corridor on the left that must run at the back of the kitchen.

'Down here are the bathrooms.'

From what I can tell, the corridors on either side of the kitchen lead to rooms and to these bathrooms. The only difference between them being that this corridor leads to the stairs whereas the other leads to the back door. I follow Gina up the steps, gripping onto the handrail as I go. I'm good but not exactly an Olympian at going up straight stairs ... never mind ones that look like cheesy triangles. There's a length of glass that runs behind the stairs. Through it, I snatch glances of the pool, the white slabs running around it and an area at the back for sitting under a cream-coloured canopy.

'This is my room. You can give me a knock at any time if you need me,' Gina says, as we reach the top of the stairs, pointing to the door straight across from us.

She leads me down the corridor, gesturing, with a timing that shows she's done this tour a thousand times before, to the doors on the left.

'These are private rooms. Only these two are for rent, though. The other ones aren't ready. We've been doing them up when we can. We're small but homely … well, that's what we aim for,' she states proudly.

I nod, wondering how often she's used that line but warmed by how she uses the word 'we' as though I'm already a part of the place.

'This is your room. You'll be sharing with the other volunteers and sometimes with guests but it's low season so, unless we get a big party, you should have the room to yourselves. At the moments it's just Hale in here,' Gina says, opening the door at the end of the corridor.

The small room essentially consists of the same bunkbeds as downstairs. They have the same lockers underneath them and curtains which can be pulled around the sides like on hospital beds.

'Ah, about time!' comes an enthusiastic female voice, her head appearing from the nearest of the lower bunks. 'Been waiting for another girl for ages.'

'Well, you should have two soon. Hale, this is Joy,' Gina

informs her with a smile. Turning to me she adds, 'You can just relax for tonight and tomorrow you'll be shown what work you're to do.'

'Thanks.'

Gina leaves the room, leaving me to stand awkwardly in the middle of it – unsure of what to do.

'Where's your stuff?' Hale asks, swinging her legs out from the bunk and giving me the once over. Her tanned skin and the hooded shape of her eyes reminds me of Gina, but her thick dark hair is dyed blue at the tips.

'Downstairs,' I say.

'Why's it down there?'

'I … I wasn't told to take it with me,' is the best reply I can think of.

'Ok,' she says slowly, looking at me a little oddly before adding, 'Pick a bed and I'll go get it.'

She bounces off her bed and out the room with an annoying amount of energy – while I stand listlessly looking around. My eyes scan the cramped room until they settle on the bed most hidden away in the corner. When Hale returns with Old Faithful, she leaves it at my feet and flounces back into her bunk, her short and slender frame sliding easily between the two.

'I wouldn't pick that one. It squeaks,' she informs me, as I head over to my corner bunk.

'Oh, ok, thanks,' I mutter, moving to the bunk opposite her.

'Are you wanting top or bottom?'

'Top,' I say. I don't know why but it seems safer somehow.

'Then I wouldn't pick that one, either. We had a drunken incident and the slats are a bit broken. We reserve that one for people we don't like.'

'This one?' I ask, pointing to the one above her.

'It's fine. Plus, you're right next to the window. The curtains don't really fit so you can lie in bed and look down to the city. It's nice at night with the lights and you get the sun in the morning.'

'Great,' I say, trying to sound enthusiastic about the impending prospect of being woken at daybreak.

I glance back to the bed with broken slats. Comfort verses sleep. Reluctantly, I choose comfort; I won't get any sleep without it.

'Only downside is you have to sleep on top of me,' Hale adds jovially, with a shrug of her shoulder and a slight tip of her head as though her head and shoulder are trying to high-five each other.

'We've only just met, you sure we're ready for that?' I say dryly, shoving my suitcase to the end of the bunk.

My eyes dart to hers, unsure of how she'll interpret my words – it's the kind of thing I'd say to Logan in jest. But even when I try, it's hard to make it sound that way now. Hale stares at me impassively, her lips pinching downwards at the ends.

'I think, with a safe word, we can handle it,' she says, smiling now. 'There's a locker under the bed for you and a shelf in the corner of each bed, too. Gina can give you a key for your locker.'

'Thanks. Where are you from?' I ask, trying to make an effort seeing as I'm going to be living with her.

'I was born in Hawaii like Gina but I moved a lot. I've lived in heaps of places.'

'Wow, that must have been … nice, to travel so much,' I say, trying to decide if it actually would be or not.

Hale shrugs dismissively and looks away, clearly not wanting to speak about it, so I quickly change the subject.

'How long have you been here?'

'A few weeks, I think. But I come here most years,' Hale

explains, straightening her legs and wiggling her fluffy-sock-covered toes. Her familiarity in the way she speaks to Gina is making more sense now.

'Is there anything I should be doing?' I ask.

'Not unless Gina asks you to do something.'

'Ok, I'll just ... sort my stuff out,' I think out loud.

I take out the things I'll need for bed tonight but other than that there's nothing for me to do.

'Hale?' I say, to get her attention from the notepad she's drawing in. 'What time does it get dark here?'

'About five.'

'Is there a shop nearby? I should probably get some food,' I say.

I'm hoping she'll freely tell me what normally happens here food wise – food is meant to be provided but it seems rude to presume given that I'm not working yet.

'There's shops everywhere.'

I resist the urge to thank her for her unhelpfulness and then, after a moment of me silently biting my tongue, she adds, 'If you go out and turn right and just keep on that road you'll come to a bigger shop, it has more options. If you go all the way to the bridge then you've gone too far.'

'Thanks,' I mutter.

I get the key for my locker from Gina, who sits crossed-legged like a skinny Buddha on the stool behind reception, as I pass her on my way outside. I follow Hale's directions and head down the street I originally walked up to get to the hostel.

Now I'm not hunting for the hostel, I pay more attention to the numerous houses around me; most of which are walled or fenced in like the hostel. The buildings themselves mostly have white walls and red-tiled roofs and are roughly the same size as the hostel, which is just on the outskirts of the city, the higher rising buildings slowly appearing amongst shorter ones as you get closer to the centre.

It's a nice area I tell myself, looking at the trees that line the empty roads, the nearly deserted streets making me all the warier of those I do meet. I hadn't noticed the mountains overshadowing part of the city until now; it's almost as though they're cupping the city, keeping it close like a protective parent.

I keep wondering how I'm meant to feel about being here. I've been good at keeping it out of my head but since Gina's comment, I can't help the thoughts, which wonder what it would be like if I weren't here alone. I let the thought flutter through my mind before swatting it away again … Reality's cruel.

After five minutes, I'm confronted with the grand Eagle Bridge – their penetrating eyes staring down at me in mockery for somehow managing to walk past the shop without noticing. Opposite the bridge, up a steep hill, is the ruin of a castle. A small but noticeable number of tourists are milling about and leaning over the ramparts to get a view of the city below them. I watch them for a moment before slowly backtracking the way I came.

I'm about halfway between the bridge and the hostel when I spot the shop. Inside, I peruse the shelves; the names, brands, language and prices utterly unfamiliar.

I wander around aimlessly, growing more and more compressed by the magnitude of the unknown. I look about me, increasingly aware of how much I stand out here. My extreme paleness appears to be a novelty to the tanned bodies around me, for their eyes bore into me as I pass them. I shouldn't be surprised.

Maltdonia isn't exactly a popular holiday destination but still I never anticipated it. I finally find what I think is porridge and a bag of nuts but I struggle to find anything I can make into a meal. All of the things I can accurately guess the contents of, by the picture on the packaging, are all the things my diet won't allow me to eat. I pause at the end of the aisle, my scant items clutched tightly in my tired arms. If nothing else, I reconcile, I can have some porridge for dinner. I'll have to make it with water seeing as I can't find milk, but that's ok, I reassure myself.

I stand at the end of the line of people waiting to pay, the 300 Maltdonian Nix note in my hand – for all I know I could be handing over £30 for my porridge and bag of nuts. My naivety in my hasty decision to come here keeps hitting me, catching the air from my lungs like a pump which won't fill.

The woman behind the till scans my items and asks me something in Maltdonian before sighing at my uncomprehending expression and tapping the screen to show me my bill. I hand over what I think is owed then take my scant items outside, glancing around me at all the people going about their lives as though the world is ordinary. Slowly, I head back towards the hostel, my mind lost in the irony that my external world now encompasses my internal one … I'm lost, alone and in a country that doesn't feel any less foreign to me than being back home.

Chapter Twenty-eight

JOY – AGE 25

Is it just me or does anyone else see the madness in me living in a hostel, in a foreign country, when:

A) I know nothing about hostels, never mind having never stepped in one.
B) I've not left my own country in over twelve years and most definitely never alone.
C) I've not shared a room since I was nine.
D) I virtually live alone … I now live, on average, with sixteen people!

Hale and I spend most of my first full day here wandering. She takes me around the new city and along the riverside I walked down when I first arrived. She explains how the intricate and ancient-looking buildings are fake. How it's a façade put onto the building's exterior, by the government, to try to draw in tourists. The buildings' new exterior explains the somewhat fake feel the new city has, like a bowl of wax apples, it's too shiny to be true. As we wander around, Hale points to paint-splattered walls and statues – the remnants of peaceful protests over what the people saw as a huge waste in expenditure.

We pause to have lunch in the main square where we're

watched over by a huge statue of an ancient mythical war hero. Afterwards she takes me over the battered bridge, which I thought looked so out of place when I arrived, that leads to the old city. I prefer it here with its small shops and merchants selling random items on the street; it feels authentic in its rustic ways. Hale ends her tour by taking me up to the castle but there's maintenance going on so we can't go inside.

Once we get back to the hostel, later that afternoon, I take a short nap under the pretence of writing an email to everyone back home. When I get up, I feel worse than I did before, my body groggy and heavy from walking in the heat. As I head downstairs towards the communal room my stomach begins to tighten; the murmur of voices growing louder and louder the closer I get to it. I hesitate as I come round the corner into the communal room and see that dinner is being served in the kitchen by Gina and Hale.

'What can I do?' I ask, taking a breath before making myself step up to the bar top.

'If I pass you things, can you put them on the table?' Gina asks distractedly, handing me a bowl of salad.

I take it from her and start my to-and-fro journey from the kitchen to the table with bowls of potatoes, chicken in tomato sauce, some vegetarian variation, bread and other things whose contents I can't even guess the name of.

The inviting smell of food seems to draw people from every room and corner of the hostel and, curious about what's been made, they all have a look to see what's on offer.

'You're welcome to join us,' Gina says, to my dismay, to each and every one of them.

I reluctantly gather more cutlery as the numbers increase. My slim frame squeezing through the growing cluster of people who have gathered and who all want to help but ultimately get in my way. I pause as I wait for one of the guests to move aside, a stack of glasses clutched tightly in my hands as the sea of people presses in around me. I hang my head momentarily and close my eyes but, when I open them again, everything seems more suffocating than it was before.

The airy communal room is so compact it seems impossible to have ever felt spacious. I try to breathe but I'm wrapped by invisible bonds. I keep holding my breath, absurdly aware that I'm sharing everyone's air and there's not enough of it. I edge my way to the table, feeling too small, feeling like even the shortest amongst them is towering over me. I set down the tower of glasses and move into the only corner of the room which isn't crammed with people.

My eyes pick out pieces of movement: Lev (another guest cum permanent resident) carrying extra chairs to the table; Gina, laughing from over the kitchen bar at something one of the guests has just said to her; Hale, holding a bowl over her head, a smile on her lips as she twirls between two guests to avoid a collision. My gaze meanders from one face to the other. Everyone's smiling happily, chatting animatedly or comfortably watching what's going on. So why am I the only one who seems so ... so ... I don't even know.

One step. One breath. One step. One breath. That's all you need I remind myself, but my mantra just feels feeble.

'Take up a seat everyone ... wherever you can find one!' Gina laughs, her face alight with the noise and the bustle as everyone does as instructed.

By the time I find my way to the table I'm forced to sit, with my arms tucked tightly into me, between two guests with another sitting unsettlingly out of sight behind me. I'm hardly in my seat before bowls of food are being passed to me, in such quick succession I can hardly keep up. I take a little bit of everything before racing to pass it on.

'See,' Lev says, pointing his fork towards me, his Russian accent drawling and thick. 'The little ones eat the most,' he says, nudging Hale who's sitting next to him.

I look down at my mound of food which I felt too uneasy to refuse.

'So what's your excuse?' Hale retorts jovially.

'I'm growing,' Lev says in mock defence. His mop of long curly hair, like his exuberant gestures, bobbing about with him. 'You're a very quiet person?' Lev says to me from across the table. He doesn't seem to say it as an insult but merely an observation.

I glance at Gina, who's watching me intently, the criteria list for her volunteers flashing through my mind – outgoing, social and I was becoming so … before. I wonder if the polite warning on the site is something she'd follow through on? She doesn't seem like the kind of person who would send someone home but, at the same time, there's something about Gina that makes me disinclined to test that.

'Jetlag. Anybody want this?' I say brightly, in a meagre attempt at compensation, holding out a bowl of the vegetarian variation.

'Me,' a guest, I can't even see, calls from up the table.

I pass it up to them but the weight of Gina's eyes seems to laden my shoulders, compressing them as though pulling them downwards, making movement far harder than it should be.

I watch as everyone passes food, switches cutlery and grabs at various things with their hands. My body presses into the back of the wooden chair, recoiling from the thought of all the bacteria and germs they're spreading to the food we're eating. I watch with revulsion as one of the guests uses their own spoon in some of the communal dishes – I instantly blacklist those bowls.

I guess they can take such things for granted; they don't have to worry about a weakened immune system or the consequences a seemingly small ailment could cause … I envy and resent their lack of necessity to care.

I gaze down at the mound of food in front of me, my body repulsed by it. I want to flee from the noise of everyone chattering, forks clattering, knives clacking, the pressure pressing upon me like a physical force. I bite the inside of my cheeks, knowing how differently I'd feel right now if the last spare chair were taken. I swallow the rough pip of loss lodged in my throat, before making myself pick up my fork – suppressing the desire to wipe it despite the lack of dirt evident upon it. I make myself eat, despite the tight knot in my stomach, for fear of being rude. With every mouthful I take, the more I think I might choke. I eat as much as I can but I can't eat nearly as much as I took.

'Your eyes are bigger than your stomach,' one guest remarks fondly when he sees me struggling.

'I'll eat it,' Lev says quickly, eagerly leaning over the table to see what's left on my plate.

'Lev,' Gina warns softly.

'Sorry,' Lev says, instantly sitting back down. 'Are you done?'

'Here,' I say, willingly handing it over to him before adding to Gina and Hale, 'It was really nice.'

'Thank you,' Gina replies, with a nod of acknowledgement. 'If you're finished, I'll show you what to do while you're on shift tonight.'

I nod, making myself smile as though I'm excited, while another loop knots in my stomach. Why on earth did I think I could do this?

'It's very easy,' Gina tells me as she leads me over to the reception desk while everyone else clears up from dinner. 'You get two types of guests. The walk-ins and the bookers. Generally, we know in advance and whoever is handing over the shift will tell you if anyone is due to arrive. However, some people book on the doorstep and then come in saying they've already booked but it's not come through the system yet, so don't worry if that happens.'

'Why do they do that?' I ask.

'They get a small discount for booking online,' she explains, pulling a thick and heavily thumbed book from under the lip on the desk.

'You ask for the guest's passport and fill in their name, DOB, birthplace, nationality, passport number and then ask how they entered the country. If they don't want to pay until they leave or if they don't have money on them to pay, then you hold their passport and lock it in the drawer here,' she says, pointing to the bottom drawer of the desk, which has a reinforced lock.

'Otherwise, they can pay when they arrive and you can give them their passport back. Make sure that they are paying in Maltdonia Nix, though – the cash tin is in that drawer and whoever is handing over the shift will give you the keys. It's vital that you keep the keys on you at all times. Don't set them down anywhere or lose them.'

I watch Gina turn to the computer, glad for the momentary reprieve in her monologue, my fingers fighting the urge to rub my reeling head.

'The password for the computer is here.' Gina points to a scrap of paper hidden away under a mug full of pens. A sheen of light, from the desk's lamp, rippling through her hair as she moves. 'To check which beds are free or which ones have been reserved for guests who've booked, you simply pull up this tab on the computer and look at the graph. Red means the bed's taken, amber means it's booked and green means it's free.'

'Right,' I mutter, my voice sounding far smaller than I want it to be.

I shift my weight from one foot to the other, trying to ease out the aching in my joints from standing stagnant.

'Then you show the guest where the kitchen and the bathrooms are, tell them to make themselves at home and show them to their room. If everyone is asleep you remind them, politely, to be as quiet as possible. You can turn on the guide lights above the door,' Gina instructs.

I nod as though I'm following everything she's saying, but my disease-ridden brain makes her words sound like they're running together into an unintelligible flow of nothing but noise.

'Other than keeping the place looking tidy, your only job is to chat to the guests, make them feel welcome at all times and to make sure that after ten they're quiet – especially when they come in at night and they've had a drink. If someone is checking out in the morning, all you need to do is ensure they've paid and stop them leaving if they haven't. If they've paid, check to make sure we don't have their passport and that they've given their locker key back if they paid for one. It's ten Nix if someone does want one and the key for each bed is in the drawer. Each number on the key is assigned to the number written on each bed.'

'Ok, great.' I can't think of a less accurate word to express what I think and feel right now but I can hardy tell her that. Something of the notion must have leaked onto my face though, for she pauses as though to assess me.

'I think, once you've settled into your first few nightshifts, we'll tell you the rest of your duties,' Gina tells me, confirming what I suspected. 'You're welcome to come to any of us, at any time, if you're unsure of anything. There's no one booked to check in so, unless we get a walk in, it should be a quiet night for you.'

'Thanks,' I say, gripping onto the outside of my thighs.

'It seems like a lot but it's very simple once you get your head around it. I'll let you know when your shift starts.'

I nod and leave her to it. Sighing silently, I make my way back to the communal room, where there's a group of people playing on the guitars and drums in the corner. Lev hands me a small drum and I try to join in but all I can think about is the fact that I haven't worked in over nine years, I'm chronically ill, in a foreign country, doing a job I have no experience of doing and how I wish I wasn't here doing it alone.

At ten o'clock, the shift is handed over to me as Hale, Lev, some other guests and I are playing cards. And, as evening deepens, guests and residents slowly slope off to bed leaving the busy hostel in a surprising state of silence.

'I'm going to bed,' Hale announces, the last one standing. She stretches her arms and legs up into the air like a starfish before letting them collapse back down to her sides. 'Oh, you're up.'

Confused, I glance around to see a smartly dressed girl, about Hale's and my age, standing in the entrance between the lobby and communal room. Her bright blond hair standing out against her bronzed skin, and yet there's something in the shade of it which makes me think that her original shade of white is as pale as mine.

'Hi,' I say a little breathlessly, as I hasten to get off the couch and head over to reception.

The girl slowly comes into the room and stops in front of the desk, her eyes glancing over every surface before they land on me.

'Are … do you have a booking?' I fluster, shaking the mouse to awaken the screen.

'No, I'm a volunteer,' she informs me curtly, as though this were obvious.

'Ah, you must be Claire,' Hale says brightly, jumping up and bouncing over to us. 'I'm Hale and this is Joy … it's her first night shift.'

Claire glances at me as though that much were evident.

'You'll still need her passport details,' Hale instructs me, even though they never asked for mine.

Claire gives me what I need and I fill her details into the book. I hand back into her perfectly manicured fingers, her passport and the key to her locker –

which volunteers get for free.

'I can take you up to our room. I'm going to bed anyway,' Hale says.

'Thanks,' I say.

'We're sharing a room?' Claire asks, askance.

Hale and I exchange a look before Hale spins on her heels and heads down the hall.

'Why don't you take the top bunk opposite ours,' I hear Hale suggest as they walk away from me.

Chapter Twenty-nine

BETH

The biggest challenges when caring for the recovering sick:

- Letting go – it's a bit like letting your child walk to school on their own for the first time … only all the usual risks and dangers are a million times higher.
- Cotton wool – similar to the above only with different context. I'm not exaggerating when I say I've spent tens of thousands of pounds, not just on raising said child but on the medical bills to keep her alive. To risk anything happening to her would be like taking an antique ornament, worth millions, and throwing it out of a plane.
- When to intervene – you know when your child's learning to be independent and you have to make yourself sit back and watch them struggle in order to let them learn … it's a lot like that. Only after spending nearly a decade as their carer, it's almost impossible not to take over.
- Living – you end up spending so much time facilitating the life of another that you forget to live your own.

It's been over a week since Joyce – Joy – left and I've still not adjusted to her departure. Each night I wander around the cottage feeling it as empty and as vast as an abandoned mansion, unnerving in its eery stillness. I wonder if this is what it felt like for Joy all these years. I've waited so long to be here alone, to have my cottage to myself, and now I'd do anything to have it full again.

Reluctantly, I shut off the TV and get to my feet. Eager for bed.

'Dog,' I call, abruptly noticing his absence.

'Do—' my voice fades away. Already, I know where he'll be.

I trudge up the stairs, my eyes instantly confirming my hunch when I see that the door to Joy's room is open. I stand in the doorway, the light from the hall falling and framing me across the floor and up her wall. Dog lies at the top of her bed, his head resting where her head should be.

'You missing her?' I say quietly.

I watch him for a moment before crossing the room to climb into bed with him.

'Me too,' I whisper, wrapping my arm around him.

I lie there, the warmth of Dog and the smell of Joy soothing the gap she's left in me.

I wake up the next day with a stiff neck and very little space on Joy's bed. It takes me a moment to understand how and why I am where I am. I smile as I sit up to examine the proportions of the bed I've slept in, amazed at how one dog can somehow manage to dominate the entire space.

I stretch, luxuriating in the knowledge that I've no rush to be anywhere. The job I was meant to be on was cancelled last night. I could easily have taken up another but I couldn't face the thought of having to arrange it. I sigh as I get to my feet, before heading downstairs where I ponder over breakfast what I'm meant to do for the next two days. After my first morbid night here alone,

I filled the gap which was consumed by Joy with work. I even started taking Dog with me so that I could walk him during my lunch breaks.

After washing up my dishes, I stand by the sink, the coolness of the tiles leaching into my toes as I inspect the kitchen with unrushed eyes. The more I look the more I see it's clean but far from immaculate. So, I hoover, I scrub, I even dust for cobwebs but that only takes me up to mid-morning. I take Dog for a good hike which takes me up to lunch and then I sit on the couch until boredom dictates that I do something. I wander through the house looking for things to do. I pause as I come back downstairs, my eyes lingering on the only room I've not entered. I reach out a hand and push at the door into Joy's second bedroom, the door slowly swinging open before me to reveal her lifeless room.

While Dog dashes into the room, my own entrance is hesitant. I take in the sofa bed, the clothes piled on the floor because there was not enough space for drawers, the box of drugs in the corner and the wall marred by her liquid medication – which I splashed up the wall while attempting to get the lid off. Now I look at it, the walls are pretty scuffed and marked – most probably from Joyce using them to help keep her upright.

I set about stripping the sofa bed, dumping the dirty sheets on the floor as I go, which Dog instantly curls up into. I tug at the stubborn mattress protector, deciding to clean it all, my body stumbling backwards as it gives way. I gasp out of shock rather than pain as my elbow hits the fireplace and knocks over an ornament, my body flinching at it breaking into countless shards on the hearth, thinking of the pain the noise will cause Joy. I straighten up a little though as I realise that Joy's not here … I can make as much noise as I want. I stare at the broken pieces around me, my mother's prized ornament now unrecognisable. She adored it ... I hated it. Joyce hated it too, she hated having them in here and I must confess when she was sullen and ill-tempered it brought me satisfaction to think of her having to look at them all day.

I pick up the next ornament, clasping it in my hand for a moment before uncurling my fingers and letting it roll off my hand. I watch it smash with a small smile of satisfaction. I tuck my hand behind the next one and simply nudge it off. One after another until there's nothing left other than their shattered remains. I glance round the room, a room which has contained nothing but misery for almost a decade now, a room which is cast in the darkness of the shadows of memories that should no longer live here.

I quickly clean up the fragments, ideas racing through my mind, before hastening to leave the house. Two hours later, I stand in some tattered old clothes inspecting the wall before me. With a smile, I turn up the volume on my old portable player before grabbing the roller next to me and, before I can stop myself, I roll a line of sunset pink onto the wall. Deeply unsure of my colour choice but nonetheless committed, I keep going. I work into the evening, my glass of wine smeared with fingerprints of paint. I paint, I drink, I dance to myself as I go. Pleased by my progress and fuelled by my booze, I call Liz and invite her round for dinner tomorrow night along with the rest of the girls.

'Including Cathy?' Liz jokes.

'Mhhh, sure,' I say, looking around my newly decorated room.

I spend the next day franticly scrubbing the skirting boards, scraping paint off places it wasn't meant to land on and rearranging the furniture. I forgot what a good space this was, I think to myself as I pause to admire my work. With the sofa bed tucked back into a sofa, the room is transformed. It's light and airy. The white table sits invitingly in the centre with the chairs around it. I pause as I consider the room, pondering for a moment before I recall what's missing.

Dog and I head out to the shed and dig out some old paintings I've been storing for the day I could reclaim the room as mine. I wipe down the frames, smiling at my charity shop finds that have been hidden for so long that I almost forgot they were there.

Once I'm content that they won't fall down, I head to the kitchen to start cooking, happily banging every cupboard door and utensil as I go, my music blaring to my heart's content. At five o'clock I head upstairs to get ready, excitement bubbling inside me as I change my clothes. I pause as I catch myself in the mirror, considering what to do with my face and hair. I pull out a pair of old straighteners which make a worrying whine as they heat up. While they do, I put on some foundation and mascara. Hesitantly, I examine myself in the mirror, oddly discontent with the feeling of the chemicals on my skin. I'm so unused to wearing makeup that I'm not sure I look like myself with it on, it almost feels garish, but by the time I straighten my hair it's too late to remove it.

'You look amazing,' Liz tells me, hugging me and then holding me at arm's length to take me in.

'Oh, thank you,' I say self-consciously, moving aside to let the others in.

'If I was doing it again, I'm not sure I'd pick that colour,' I confess to them, an hour later as we sit down to eat in the dining room.

'I like it, it's very you,' Liz says, admiring my efforts.

'What – unconventional?' Jossey laughs.

I lift my glass to cheers myself.

'Is that a Kemp Co original?' Cathy asks, her eyes fixated on my newly mounted painting.

'It is,' I say smugly.

'But they're so rare, how – how did *you* get one?'

'Oh, he gifted it to my great-grandfather,' I lie, winking at the other girls.

'Really?' Cathy says, drawing out the word in her wonderment.

'No, I got it from the charity shop,' I laugh.

'Oh ... oh, I don't ever go into those places,' she confesses. 'Maybe I should if they sell such collectables.'

'How's Joy getting on?' Liz asks, changing the subject. 'I can't believe she's abroad. She's come so far.'

'I know, I can't believe it either. She's fine I think ...' I say awkwardly, taking a sip of wine. 'I'm trying not to message her too much. I want to give her space to enjoy herself.'

'Ah, of course, it's so hard to do that though, isn't it?' Jossey chips in, with an understanding nod of the head. 'I remember when James went abroad for the first time ... I pestered him relentlessly.'

I take another gulp of wine, not wanting to admit that we haven't spoken since she messaged to say she'd arrived. I keep picking up my phone to message her but something stops me. The longer she's away, the more I question myself. I can't deny anymore that there's a large part of me that doesn't want to let her go, that wants to keep her where she is for fear of being alone. If I'm brutally honest, I'm scared, I'm scared of not being needed or wanted anymore. My life has revolved around her for so long that losing her would be to lose myself too. My very purpose in life would be gone. While she's been getting better, she's been evolving and discovering who she is and yet I've stayed still. She and I were swaying to the same dance and now she's doing her own and I'm left fighting the desire to pull her back to the dance we're so used to doing together.

'So, whose turn is it to host next?' Liz asks, bringing me out of my reveries.

Chapter Thirty

JOY – AGE 25

I wriggle into my shorts, regretting my choice of denim as I struggle to get them on within the scant privacy of my curtained upper bunk. I lie back on my bed for a moment, waiting for the weary sensation in my limbs to settle. I sigh into the silence. Getting dressed is more taxing than one of those workout videos. I heave myself up and carefully make my way down the ladder of my bunk, pausing at the bottom, my limbs feeling hollow.

I've been off nightshift for days now but I still feel like my body's catching up from the exhaustion of getting here.

Hale, Claire and I take it in turns to work the nightshift – three nights on and three nights off. Given the low season, the work is far from laborious. There are two other members of staff who are both called Marty. You'd think that might make it easier to remember, only one of them is nicknamed Smarty and for the life of me I can't remember which. Gina, I've learned, has a second job which takes her out of the hostel most days and so Marty, Smarty, Hale, Claire and I are trusted to take charge.

Despite my initial unease, within a week or so of being here I've somehow settled into the routine of hostel living. My phone has become my saviour though; I've taken to writing everything down in it, saving me the mortification of having to ask the same questions because I constantly forget the answers. To begin with I could see them giving me odd looks as though wondering if I'm simple but, as time's gone on, I somehow seem to have proven them wrong and they now view my forgetfulness as an endearing personality quirk rather than the degrading, humiliating danger to discovery that I perceive it as.

I crouch next to Hale's unmade and uninhabited bed before opening my locker and pulling Old Faithful out from its depth. I glance towards Claire's bed, my eyes surveying the closed curtain around it and conclude that if I can't see her then she can't see me.

I open the already unzipped lid of Old Faithful, cringing at the sharp rustle of the heavy plastic bag which contains all my smaller bags of meds. As quietly as I can, I begin opening the clear zip-lock bags. Each weighty bag holds two months' worth of different tablets.

I pick out what I need for today and put them in an empty bag, ready for later, before swallowing my morning tablets with some bottled water I keep in my trunk. As quietly as I can, I bury the heavy bag, like a pick and mix of drugs, at the bottom of my case before pushing Old Faithful back into the locker. Despite my gentleness, the metal locker door still clatters and shudders as I close it and push the padlock shut with a snap.

I twist around, glancing up to Claire's top bunk. The realisation hitting me as hard as the nausea which drops and swirls in my stomach like cement in a mixer. Slowly, I look around to the bottom bunk in the corner to see Claire watching me from the gap in her curtain. Our eyes lock and hold each other like an accident you can't look away from, before she pulls the curtain tightly around her bed … obscuring her from view. I look down at my hands and the white powder still coating my palms, cursing my stupid memory and the fact she moved bunks two nights ago.

I head downstairs, my legs abruptly feeling far weaker than they did just moments before. In the kitchen, I check how full the kettle is before switching it on, watching with unfocused eyes as the gradual burble of the ancient contraption comes to life. I slowly draw myself from my daze to put away the dishes on the dryer, as though trying to prove to myself my helpfulness here. I even wipe down the stained and crumb-smattered worktops.

'You ok?' Hale asks, from the couch opposite the kitchen bar top, her voice rough and detached sounding, her body curled up and buried under blankets – we're allowed to doze during nightshift … they call it a fox's sleep because you're never truly asleep.

'I'm fine,' I mutter, occupying myself by preparing the cups. 'Busy night?'

I've learned conversation is a constant requirement here. Being social, I guess, is the whole ethos behind hostels after all. Besides, it's not like her to leave the place in a mess, but she doesn't respond.

I glance at Hale, who's curled up on the sofa watching me with bleary eyes.

'What's wrong? Are you sick?'

'I'm angry,' she says, her voice cracked with exhaustion.

'… At me?' I ask hesitantly, pausing as I scoop out tea leaves from the jar, taken aback by her candour.

'No,' Hale states, her reply as fierce as the growing rumble of the kettle.

When it clicks off, I pour the hot water into the pot; the loose leaves swirling around the glass pot, like snow in a globe, while I try to think of an appropriate reply.

'What's happened, then?' I ask.

Pouring the tea into two cups – one with milk and the other without – and heading into the sitting room, I hand a heavy-eyed Hale the cup without milk before sitting on the other end of the couch. I take it as a good sign that she curls up her knees and sits up to make room for me. She holds up the corner of the blanket she's tucked herself beneath so I can join her.

She sips her black tea as though in need of it to bring her from the depth, her dark hair scrunched up at the back so that the blue tips lie halfway up her neck.

My reluctant lips smile at one of the guests as he stumbles past us on the way to the kitchen. I wait for Hale to say something to him, to strike up a conversation so I don't have to but she doesn't.

'Good night?' I ask him eventually.

'Yeah, wasn't bad actually. This for anyone?' he asks, pointing at the pot.

'Help yourself.'

'Thanks. I hope we didn't keep you up too late,' he says, a little shamefacedly, to Hale.

She looks at him for a moment and I can almost hear the debate between what she wants to say and what she must say going through her mind.

'No problem,' she says dryly.

'I'll try to get them to behave a bit more,' he says, before doing the walk of embarrassment back to his room with his mug of tea; to wait for his friends (who I presume are still in a drunken stupor – as they have been every morning since they arrived here three days ago).

'His friend puked on the front door, down himself, in the hall and in his bed,' Hale tells me, once the dorm room door clicks shut.

'Classy,' I say tersely.

'I couldn't even change his sheets because there're no clean ones.'

'That can't be right,' I reply.

Hale looks at me like I'm an idiot so I rephrase.

'How are there no sheets?'

'Because Claire's been on shift the last three nights.'

'Yeah,' I say, dismissing this piece of information, which I already know.

'Well ...' Hale says, as though waiting for me to catch on. 'She's not done any washing in the last three nights and we had all those people leave on the same day, remember ... we have nothing clean. I've been looking after Mr Puker while his mates were passed out and washing bed sheets all night. Only we've run out of places to hang the wet ones.'

I take a long sip from my cup, unsure of what to say or how to react, so I ask the only question which strikes me. 'What's she been doing each night?'

'Sleeping.'

Hale and I sit and sip our tea, both of us in silent contemplation.

The sad thing is that Claire makes me look good in comparison. Still, I fidget where I sit, wondering how it must look in a stranger's eyes to have seen what she saw me doing. Someone taking a few tablets is innocent enough, but I was taking handfuls.

I wrap my free arm around myself. I can't stand the idea of them knowing the truth. I'm not stupid. Hiding my illness doesn't make it go away, but it's been so long since I've been able to just be. As soon as a person knows you're sick it's always there, that knowledge subconsciously influencing them. Here, it's not the thing that defines me and I'd do anything to keep it that way.

I hold out my hand to Hale. 'Here, give me the keys and go to bed.'

'Thanks, but there's only an hour left and I need to explain what's happened. I don't want them thinking it was me.'

'I'll tell them,' I offer, but she just shakes her head.

'I'm too annoyed to sleep,' she sulks, before adding with irritation. 'You notice how she disappears every day, too. She's never about, never helps show the guests around the city or chats to them. Never helps tidy or clean the place.'

'Yeah,' I mutter guiltily.

Twenty minutes later, the one I think is Marty appears for his shift, wishing us a good morning as he comes in the door before reassessing.

'Or not?' he says cautiously, eyeing Hale.

'The pot's not long made if you want a cup,' I tell him.

Marty steps gently towards the kitchen, assessing if it's tea or coffee. He always reminds me of a robin – always curious and forever hesitant. He's a lot more reserved than Smarty, shorter and far slighter in build too (although that's not particularly hard, given that everyone is smaller and slighter than Smarty).

'Was it a busy night?' he asks, his quiet voice always calming and yet I'd be hesitant to call him a pushover.

'I'll explain once Gina's down,' Hale decides.

Ten minutes later, I sit at the table eating my breakfast of porridge, honey and cinnamon, while pretending not to eavesdrop as Hale explains to Marty and Gina what's happened. Although I can't hear what's being said, it's clear from the discontent on each of their faces that they're not impressed. After a time, Hale disappears to bed and the normal routine of paperwork, sweeping, mopping, helping guests and tidying is resumed. I sit and read for a while, pausing only when Claire appears from upstairs and heads into the kitchen. I glance over in time to watch Marty lean back on the reception chair to say something to Gina, who's sitting in the office. A moment later she appears in the doorway.

'Claire, once you've made your drink would you come and have it in here with me?' Gina asks lightly.

'I'm about to go out,' Claire states.

'This won't take long,' Gina says pointedly.

'Sure,' Claire replies, like a hare unaware of the snare.

I watch Claire slowly make her coffee and head to the office, the door of which is, for the first time when someone's in it, closed behind her.

'Do you have the list of things you need picked up today?' I ask Marty from across the room.

'Mhh, yes but Gina was writing it.' He glances at the closed door. 'I can go in and get it if you want it now?'

'... I can wait.'

Five minutes later, Claire reappears. She pauses behind reception as though unsure of what do to with herself.

'Ow, sorry,' Marty hastens to say, as he pushes his chair back and nearly bashes into her.

Claire jumps back, scurrying out from behind the desk and

knocking over a stack of information books about Maltdonia – sending them fleeing across the floor, her normal composure shattered as she stoops to pick them up.

'I'll get it,' Marty offers gently, instantly sliding off his seat as though helping's never a consideration and simply a response.

I watch, unmoving, that instinct long lost to me … You learn the hard way to conserve energy wherever you can – even at the expense of others.

Claire stands, her eyes doing a sweep of possible exits before heading past me to the back door.

I know I should ask her if she's ok – possibly I should even follow her to make sure – but for some reason I can't get my body or mouth to move. Carrying the weight of my own scars is heavy enough without carrying someone else's too. I look down at my hands, which were forever extended to others. They could never see a hurt soul go without consoling. I wonder at what point I lost that. I can carry off a good facade of empathy when I need too but underneath I quickly grow bored of the insignificance and repetition of peoples' woes, of their pathetic ability to feel everything – it only ever sentences them to be damned by their own emotions.

I used to think there was strength in feeling nothing but I envy them now. To find such emotional importance on such impermanent things. To be so impassioned and feeling towards something you hardly have a connection to or control over seems so dangerous to me now and yet I long to feel that alive.

I glance up as Gina appears, the movement from the corner of my eye drawing me from my reveries.

'Marty said you were waiting for the list. Don't worry if you can't get everything,' she says, putting the list on the table before me. 'Thanks, Joy.'

'Gina,' I say, as she turns to walk away.

She pauses, her head tipped to one side.

'I'll take Hale's shift tonight.'

Gina nods. 'I'm sure she'd be grateful.' She smiles, pauses and then pulls out the chair next to me. 'How are you finding things here?' she asks, sitting down beside me.

'Good,' I reply. What else can I say?

'I know … it must be tough at times so if you ever need a moment, you're welcome to take it,' she offers.

I look down at my empty bowl, my insides squirming. The context may be different but this is precisely what I didn't want.

'I'm fine,' I assure her, leaning back in my chair.

'Ok,' she says softly, her gentle eyes apprising me. 'It would be a great help if you could spend a bit more time with the guests. Just ensuring they feel included here and answer any questions they have about the city.'

'Course,' I say mutedly.

I watch her get to her feet and walk away, knowing that my lacklustre involvement here is nothing but disappointing to her. It's not like I don't do everything asked of me, I think to myself, clutching the watch on my wrist. I think about the way Hale and the two Martys get so involved and impassioned with the guests – treating them like long-lost friends. I stare at my fingers, which are fiddling with the watch strap. I'm not sure I even want to be here, but I know for certain that I don't want to be home.

Chapter Thirty-one

JOY – AGE 25

The things hostel life quickly teaches you:

1) Small talk – when you're housebound and don't ever speak to anyone new … you swiftly lose all social capabilities and niceties. Living in a hostel, however, you quickly transform from a stuttering stump of a speechless fool into the master of small talk. The trick is getting guests to talk about something they're passionate about … then you can sit back and pretend to listen.

2) Sharing – when you're sick, you hoard everything! You don't do it to be selfish but, let's face it, it's not as though you can nip to the shops to get a replacement. In a hostel, however, everyone shares everything and if it's lying around it's open to anyone.

3) Hygiene – what hygiene? You'd think, given that I used to go weeks … ok months, without washing that it wouldn't bother me but, now I'm well enough to wash, I hate the feeling of being dirty. I've learned that what I hate even more is the feeling of someone else's dirty body being in proximity to mine. Also … well, let's just say having a heightened sense of smell is not always a good thing.

4) Locks – after having doctors constantly strip you down inside and out … you either become hyper conservative or don't give a flying rat's ass. Apparently, there's a certain type of hostel goer who feels the same but, just because you're happy to show it, doesn't mean we want to see it. Said people also don't bother with closed doors, curtains or locks! If in doubt … avert your eyes!

5)..Drunksitting – you get three types of drunk guests: the frustrated and annoyed ones who've fallen out with their travel companion; the happy and affectionate; and the sad and weeping. All are noisy and all come in just when you're falling off to sleep.

That afternoon, Hale, Lev and I sit on the floor of our dorm room upstairs, an assortment of fruit juices, milk, crisps, nuts, sweets, a selection of things that remain a mystery and just about every chocolate-covered item Lev could find lies between us – the spoils of our day's discovery.

After watching Claire come back inside this morning with puffy eyes and a dark demeanour, I decided I couldn't risk not making more of an effort.

So, I went with Lev in the hunt for some fancy art pens. His company is effortless and I knew it would look good for me to be seen socialising with guests – even if it's just Lev. During our search we discovered a huge shopping centre with a massive food store. After the scant selection in the small shops nearby, our discovery was like finding a treasure trove and Lev eagerly stocked up while I collected random items just to be involved in his excitement. Neither of us considered the long hike back to Ohana until we had made our purchases and carried them out into the bright sunlight.

Tired, sweating, with arms and backs aching and with the hostel thankfully quiet, we headed upstairs to find Hale lounging on her bed after failing to sleep off her traumatic nightshift.

'Try this,' Lev says, handing me my own bag of crisps which he's opened and is sharing round.

I take a few crisps out of the bag and munch on them, my nose pinching at the strange taste.

'What's that meant to be?' I ask, as Hale laughs at the look on my face.

'I don't know,' Lev says, shaking the bag at me. His Russian accent still takes me by surprise. 'Take more, you'll like them eventually.'

'Eventually being the pertinent word,' I point out dryly, before adding to a brow-wrinkled and clearly confused Lev, 'Important.'

Lev nods in understanding but nonetheless takes my hand and gently turns my palm upwards; shaking a mound of the disgusting flavoured crisps into my hand.

Lev has been at Ohana for longer than I have and as far as I can tell he has no plans to leave anytime soon. To pay his way, he draws and sells his work in the park nearby – hence the hunt for the fancy pens, but I suspect Gina often lets him stay for free. I fail to see the artistic appeal of his work but it seems to sell well enough.

We chat about nonsense subjects, like their tattoos and the meaning behind each one and how the ones which cover Lev and part of Hale are so vibrant in colour compared to the ones I see back home. We speak about the guests, about the countless countries they've both been to, about how cheap everything is here and just about anything that pops into their heads.

Most of what's said is pointless, inconsequential, a waste of expended energy but I go along with it – it's part of my conditions in staying here, I remind myself. I try to keep up but my laughter always comes a little later than theirs and ends a little too soon. Like a jigsaw piece, I know the reactions are right for the expected space but they need forcing into place. My facial muscles hurt from trying to smile. Fake it until you feel it, I tell myself, just fake it until you feel it.

I try to stretch out my burning shoulders without them seeing. It's as if someone has soldered the blades together, my body stiff and my joints tired. While I try to subtly stretch, I watch Hale and Lev, chatting and laughing so animatedly, without a stress in the world. Life here seems so simple for everyone else, so easy and relaxed … a contradiction to everything inside myself.

I struggle to align my thinking to theirs. Everything I do back home has to have a purpose, a reason and a visible outcome, otherwise the exertion of it equals a waste but here these people do things on a whim … just because they want to, just because it's fun. I could never sustain that kind of liberty but I want to.

I watch as Lev pulls back his mop of unruly hair and tries to tuck it behind his ears … ultimately failing yet again.

'Do you want Joy and me to cut it off?' Hale offers, after his sixth attempt to tame his hair.

'My hair?' he asks and she nods. 'No, no, only my mother cut my hair.'

'We can tell,' I add and he shoves me playfully, making my mound of uneaten and strange tasting crisps spill into the floor. I look at the mess before adding with mock sorrow, 'How sad, now I can't eat them.'

'We have more,' Hale says, throwing the bag at me.

'They're good now?' Lev asks, as Hale crunches down on the

last bit of crisp in her palm before conceding that the taste grows on you.

I'm refusing some of Lev's copious supply of chocolate when the door to our room is knocked upon and opened by Gina.

'What's this?' she asks brightly, eyeing up our stash of food with an amused smile.

'We're having an indoor picnic,' Hale informs her, uncurling her legs and stretching them out before tucking one back under her.

'Want some?' Lev asks, handing her some chocolate-coated cheese bites.

'Mhh,' Gina murmurs, looking unconvinced.

She steps further into the room to get a better view of the selection, her eyes roaming over the stash. 'No, but I'd take one of those if one's going.'

Lev hands her the chocolate bar she's eyeing up.

'I've just heard that there's a local band playing tonight. Whichever of you aren't on shift, I'd be glad if you wanted to come. I think a lot of the guests will be wanting to go,' Gina tells us, unwrapping her chocolate bar.

'I'm on shift,' Hale says, unenthusiastically.

'I was going to work tonight for you,' I tell her.

Hale opens her mouth to protest but Gina cuts her off.

'That's right. Well, you can join us until your shift starts if you'd like,' Gina tells me. 'Claire, would you like to come?'

'I don't think so,' Claire says, as she comes into the room behind Gina and picks her way over our food hoard, which somehow spread its way across the room, before collapsing into her bunk and turning away from us.

I glance to Gina, who's watching Claire with pondering eyes, her head tilted, as though some great question were running through her mind. Her gaze darts to me and holds me steadfast. I want to flinch away from her stare, which strips me bare, but I don't. I sit stock still, years of self-restraint in the face of needles and probes finally coming in handy.

After a moment, I relent and look away, my eyes studying the groves in the floor. I can still feel her eyes upon me as though peeling back my skin to see that my smiles aren't real, that my laughter is forced and my interest in her guests is underlined with indifference.

Her gaze makes me feel like a fake. A liar. I laugh and joke like I'm the same as everyone else but I'm not. She sees I'm broken and destroyed and I don't know what way is up and what way's down. Yet I can't stop myself from performing this act that everything's fine. I don't know how else to do this; how else do you present yourself to the world when you feel next to nothing? If you show them the truth there'd soon be no one left to show it to – I learned that lesson the hard way and they hardly learned anything at all. I don't look up as Gina reminds us to keep the dorm tidy, in case we need to share the room with guests, before quietly shutting the door behind her.

I listen as Hale and Lev debate the merits of the biscuit they're sharing but their words seem distant now. I clasp the outside of my thighs, Gina's piercing gaze like a pin to my illusion, the cold hollow world inside me now fighting to fully embrace my external one.

I wrap my arm around myself, unsure of how you're meant to tell the world that you feel dead inside when you're supposed to be happy and grateful for being alive when others aren't. Because, how can you be sad when you're so much better than you were? But people don't see that all that does is emphasise how bad things were in the first place. It's one thing to survive this disease but it's another thing to survive in its aftermath. I never foresaw that fighting for a reason to live would be so much harder than fighting for your life.

I listen as Hale and Lev chat about their friends back home and I think how lucky they are. Because, if you're sick and you were lucky enough to have supportive people in the first place, then those people are probably fading just about now, just when you need them the most ... because they think you don't need their support anymore because the danger of death is gone, they think you're ok, and you're not, you're going through hell, only you're hiding it ... because you don't count the damage during the storm, you do that afterwards, and it's only then that you fully see the depth of destruction that changes your very soul.

'You ok ... Joy, hey, you all right?' Hale ask, cutting through my thoughts, both her and Lev staring at me.

'Yeah,' I say, smiling brightly. 'I'm good.'

I glance at them, genuine smiles and relaxed gestures ... I long so much to be like them.

Chapter Thirty-two

JOY – AGE 25

That evening, Gina, Hale, Marty and Lev take most of the guests to hear the local bands play.

Gina tried to persuade me to come until my shift starts but I told her I didn't mind staying behind to keep an eye on the boozy boys who are staying at the hostel; besides, I need to call home and say hi to everyone anyway. Both excuses are a lie. I've not spoken to Aunt Beth since I messaged to say I'd arrived and I'd far rather go to the gig but I'm already too tired as it is.

I call goodbye as I watch them leave. Their bodies dressed smartly, their voices lively with anticipation.

I wander round the empty communal room, strangely content to be working rather than joining their revelry, my fingers subconsciously tracing the rim of your watch on my wrist. I quickly let my hand fall to my side, scolding myself … the past is painful.

I glance once more around at the near empty communal room before heading into the back room, behind reception, to the mountain of washing awaiting me.

The small room contains a filing cabinet, a desk that consumes the hopes and dreams of anyone trying to find anything on it, an old and discoloured washing machine with a broken handle, a broken drier, cupboards for laundry and finally a door at the other end which leads to a fenced-off section of garden – where posts have been driven into the ground and are attached together with plastic string for washing to be hung on.

I sigh at the sight of the overflowing baskets, but in truth I revel in the task of shoving everything into the machine, of the attempt to get it to work each time without it breaking as thrilling as Russian roulette. Then taking the washing in and folding it, putting it away, hanging out the next load. It should be monotonous but I like how it numbs my mind.

Other than the group of lads who caused Hale such trauma last night, the hostel is virtually empty. A few guests appear every so often but most are either out or sleeping in their dormitories. I clean up the kitchen, check all the toilets are clean, that the handtowels are dry and that there's plenty of toilet roll. Then I head back to the sitting room to see if there's anything else I can do. When I discover there's not, I sit at reception and check for the second time if anyone is due to be checked-in tonight.

'What's the string on the roof for?' the lad who apologised on behalf of his mates this morning asks, as he comes into the communal room and sits himself down on the couch.

'The different colours point to different activities,' I say, pausing in my tidying of the desk to explain. 'There's a colour chart on the wall, so if you follow the red string it takes you to the DVDs, if you follow the blue one it takes you to card and board games, the yellow one takes you to the instruments and … so on.'

'Huh, that's pretty smart. Never seen that in a hostel before.'

'Have you stayed in a lot?'

'Not really, but I've been to a fair few,' he tells me.

'Where are you from?' I ask, my small talk seamless.

'Rotterdam,' Mr Apologetic tells me.

We chat for a while about each other's countries until his two mates decide to join him. I listen half-heartedly as they discuss their plans for the night.

'You want to come?' the other lad asks who, from Hale's description, I suspect to be Mic Puker.

'Thanks, but I'm on night shift.'

'You work here?' Mic Puker asks in surprise.

'No, I'm hanging out behind reception for fun,' I reply bluntly, before remembering myself and adding less sarcastically. 'I'm volunteering and I get my food and board in exchange.'

'Auh, smart,' he remarks, before holding up his bottle of wine and asking, 'Want some?'

'I'm fine, thanks,' I automatically say. Drinking is only allowed on nights out.

With nothing left to do at reception, I resign myself to reading my book on the couch, while keeping an eye on the three lads as they bustle around in preparation for leaving. Before too long though, all three of them are in the communal room finishing off their bottles. Their conversation and laughter grow louder with each swig, making it impossible to concentrate.

'Definitely can't come?' Mr Apologetic asks, refilling his glass.

'Tempted but can't,' I say, my lie then covered by a truth.

'Sure you don't want any?' he asks.

I go to say no but pause.

'… Actually, yeah, I'll take a glass,' I say, downing the water left in my glass and leaning over to hand it to him, the grin on my face mirroring theirs as, for once, I do what I want and not just what I'm allowed.

'Go on, join us out,' Mr Apologetic tries again, filling up my glass with wine before nudging his silent sidekick.

The third guy shoves Mr Apologetic's elbow away from him and sits up a little straighter, rubbing his weary face with both hands.

'Next time. Have fun though,' I tell him, before adding to Mic Puker, '… within reason.'

'You heard about that, huh,' Mic Puker says, with little embarrassment, downing the last of his drink.

'What happens in the hostel stays in the hostel … for *all* to hear.'

'I'll try to behave tonight,' Mic Puker adds.

'I think we both know that won't happen,' I reply pointedly.

'Don't worry, I'll keep them under control,' Mr Apologetic adds, slapping Mic Puker and Mic Sleepy, who still looks broken from the night before, on the back of the shoulders and giving them a good shake.

'What are your plans? I saw that you're checking out soon?'

'Yeah, so we're going to travel round the island, see some of the sights before our flight home,' Mr Apologetic tells me, as his broken friend slides a little further down the couch.

'So, you're not going to spend your entire holiday drunk?' I say, lifting my glass in mock cheers to the idea.

'Probably!' Mic Puker says cheerfully.

'Do you get to explore the island or are you stuck here the entire time?'

'No, we can go off for a few days if we want,' I explain, my glass cradled between my hands.

'Are you *going* to go off?' Mr Puker asks, stretching his arms above his head and almost slopping his drink over Mic Sleepy.

'Yeah, of course, we're just short of volunteers at the moment,' I say, taking a large gulp of wine.

Even as the words leave my lips, I know it's a lie. I won't be leaving here to travel, my body's struggling to withstand what I'm already asking from it but, somehow, I don't begrudge that as much as I thought I would.

'Nice, make sure you do,' Mr Apologetic says brightly, his words beginning to take on a slurring quality, while Mic Puker looks away sceptically.

'Will you still be on shift when we get back?' Mr Apologetic asks, getting to his feet.

'Probably.'

'Blooming heck, right, see you later then. Finish off what's left if you want,' he says, pointing to his second bottle of wine, which lies half empty. 'Come on, let's go,' are his parting words as he rallies his mates to get up and head out the hostel – leaving me in the eerie echo of my own silence.

I sit with the stillness. A sound once so normal to me now cradles a weight I can't stand to hold. I look around the communal room, my eyes tracing the curve of the bar, the table and the chairs tucked neatly around it. I pick up the guys' glasses and bottles that they forgot to clear away and wash them in the sink, watching as the soap bubbles run down their sides as I sit them on the drainer. I slowly dry and put them away – simply for something to do. Standing in the kitchen, alone and engulfed in stillness, with no one here whose buoyancy I can bounce off, I can feel myself deflating from the inside out. Without the distraction of others, there's nothing to fend off the darkness inside me.

I clutch Logan's watch on my wrist as a piercing chill ripples throughout my body. I stand there, not knowing what to do other than watch as the minutes tick by until all three hands of the clock unite at midnight. I stare, unblinking, as the second-hand ticks past. The communal room around me blurring before me, I close my eyes to shut it out but memories flash through me. This day last month my life changed forever once more. I was never meant to be here alone. My chest heaves for air which doesn't want to be consumed, the hostel's pungent scent of cinnamon and fruit suffocating. I shake my head, trying to stop what's building within me but I can't.

I hurry around the kitchen and down the corridor to the back door, the cool evening air hitting me as I stagger over the threshold into the back garden. I walk with deadened legs to the pool and stare down at the stars reflected on its surface – so perfect and without distortion. I sink to my knees, the slabs rough against my bare legs. I want to slip beneath the water's surface and scream until I contain no air. I want to swim amongst the peaceful stars, to absorb their tranquillity. I want to feel something other than these sudden extremes of deadness and raw reaction. I run from one to the other … unsure which one is safest, unable to handle either.

I examine my hands, the garden around me. I don't know any more what's real and what's not. What's made up and what's true. It shocks me sometimes when I pick something up and discover it has substance. It's like I'm playing a role, but this person isn't me and I don't know how to get Joy back or how to keep her.

I shake my head, trying to disrupt the thoughts that claw at my mind. I lean over, clutching my head with my hands. I don't know how to do this. I know how to be a sick person but I don't know how to live in the in between of being neither healthy nor dying. I never thought that getting better would be the hardest part of being sick.

All these strangers, constantly around me, wanting to talk to me and spend time with me and to be my friend but I don't know how to be theirs – for almost ten years I've only ever been something someone visited for ten minutes twice a year. You think it's a skill you'd never lose but that's a lie. I don't know how to be a friend or how to make one. I don't know what makes a good friend or what signals a bad one. I'm socially inept. I watch guests go out on dates and yet I don't even know what to do on one. Everyone thinks these things are instinctual but they're learned, subconsciously, over teenage heartbreaks and awkward dinner dates during uni and mistaken nights out. I don't know how far things should go or how I'm meant to feel. I have been plunged from being a child into being an adult and everyone expects me to be normal, to know what to do but I don't. I don't fit the body that I'm in but I can't escape it.

I hold onto your watch, hating you for pulling me from my slumbers, for showing me a world I forgot existed. You made me start to feel alive again and then you plunged me back into the darkness from which you found me ... and all of it and none of it is your fault. I lower myself onto the edge of the pool, daring myself to slide into its depths. I sit on the edge, my bare feet and legs slipping into the cold water ... scattering the stars.

Chapter Thirty-three

JOY – AGE 25

I sit on one of the white plastic sun loungers near the open back door, careful to keep an ear open for anyone who gets up and needs to be checked-out, a blanket, from my makeshift bed on the couch, draped over me to stave off the early morning chill. My book lies open, split down the middle, between my thighs. I had planned to come out here to read and I did for a while but without the bustle of hostel life, my mind wonders into places unwanted. My eyes glazed over the words, seeing but refusing to acknowledge their meaning … rendering reading redundant.

The colours of the rising sun, on the surface of the pool, hold my gaze as though hypnotising me. It's a sight I shouldn't be able to see; each night the pool is meant to be covered over and it's not opened until mid-morning but the mechanism for the cover jammed so the pool remains unobscured. The hostel has superseded all my scant expectations of what a hostel would be but there are things like this which reaffirm its identity. Like the tower for the flying fox, which sits at the end of the pool, nearest the house, also out of use and taped off because the water's too shallow to jump from it safely, or lamps whose wires are coming away from the switch and taped to prevent electrocution.

Once the sun settles into the sky and the usual colours of the day are set, I get up with reluctant legs and head inside. Dumping my book on the desk, I head into the back room.

I check the washing machine is definitely finished before opening it and pulling out its contents into the basket below. I made the mistake of not double-checking the first time I was charged with this duty, resulting in a torrent of water cascading out of the machine, down my legs and all over the floor.

'Look, your waters have broken,' Hale had said with glee.

My lips curve up weakly at the memory as I heave the heavy basket up onto my hip and head outside to hang up the sheets.

I put a clip at each end of the sheet before pausing to look at the sea of white all around me, fluttering in the breeze, like white waves in an ocean. I long to be washed away.

I look up sharply, at the squeak of trainers on the floor inside, to see Gina coming to a stop in the doorway.

'How was your shift?' she asks, dressed for her morning run.

Unless some unfortunate soul has an even more unfortunate flight time, Gina is usually the first to be up in the morning.

'It was good,' I report, throwing a mattress cover over the line.

'The boys get away ok this morning?'

'I got them up in time.'

'That was good of you,' Gina says, sounding pleased.

I simply shrug.

After Mic Sleepy returned back to the hostel at three in the morning and dissolved into tears on my shoulder over his ex-girlfriend, while the rest of his mates were enviously unaware, having crashed out in the dorm room, I took pity on them and woke them up in time to get their bus.

It's strange how people become a part of the hostel. I didn't think I'd notice their absence but you feel the gulf of some guests' departure more than others.

'Good! I'll see you later then,' Gina says with a smile. She turns as though to go but she pauses and turns back, her trainers squeaking sharply on the floor of the back room. 'I almost forgot. We have a surprise for you later.'

I pause mid-sheet spread, not sure how to react.

'What kind of surprise?' I settle for curiosity tinged with apprehension.

She just smiles happily as she puts her headphones into her ears, giving a brief wave as she heads out for her morning run.

I stare after her before numbly clipping the last sheet onto the line, an uncomfortable feeling settling into my stomach, which I think resembles dread.

I sit and drink a herbal tea with Hale and Lev while they eat their breakfast – waiting for one of the Martys to take over the next shift from me. The whole time Hale and Lev drop hints at every opportunity about my surprise; speaking about it to each other as though I'm not there. I know they're doing it in jest but it makes me want to pour their porridge down them. As soon as Smarty turns up, apologising for being late, I hand him the keys and go up to bed, my body and brain weary from my night of involuntary counselling.

Despite the warmth of the day already heating the room, I curl into a ball under the light blanket in an attempt to try to smother the chill living in my bones. In desperation, I put a clean sock over my eyes to block out the light, the music from my headphones gently drowning out the noise of people moving and chatting animatedly below me. I lie there, waiting for the oblivion of sleep.

'I'm going out. Do you need anything?' I ask Smarty a few hours later, standing in the doorway of the office having given up on any hope of sleep.

'Hmmm,' he pauses while folding a pillow case, a pensive look on his face. 'I don't think so. No.'

'Ok, see you in a while,' I say, turning to leave.

'Are you excited for your surprise?' he asks, halting me in my tracks, his Maltdonian accent one I'm slowly getting accustomed too.

'Yeah, Gina told me all about it. I can't wait,' I say with what I hope is enthusiasm, watching his face freeze slightly.

Smarty's tall body leans forward a little, his long face quizzical. I don't think he or the other Marty are much older than Hale or me, which almost makes our little team all the better.

'I think you're fishing in a puddle,' he says, throwing a pillowcase at me which, to my amazement, I actually catch. 'Nice try. Gina's not told anyone.'

'So that's why Hale and Lev weren't making any sense this morning,' I say.

'Are you on nightshift tonight?' he asks quickly as I throw the pillowcase back to him. It lands on his head, draping his dark buzz cut of hair like a nun's habit.

'No, Claire is,' I say, smiling at the pillowcase, which he's made no attempt to remove.

'Ok, ok, see you later,' he tells me, giving a humble bow which makes me smile.

I head to the old city, a labyrinth of shops and houses, with slopping walls and uneven roofs, wooden framed windows and doors with steps so rotten you think you'll fall through them. Countless side roads separated off from the main one like crooked fingers with uneven pavements; worn smooth and slippery by the thousands of feet that have walked upon them. The smell of roasted nuts, being cooked at the sides of the road, pungent in the air around me.

Come lunch time, queues of people will stand outside the windows of tiny shops, which sell their delicacy out of one room. The small cafés with their outside seating which make you feel like you're sat at sea, frozen at the peak of a wave, as you balance yourself on the stumped legs of stools and upside-down crates placed on the steep streets. The thin pallet tables covered in cloth. Hale and I once sat and drank tea here. While we drank our exotic tea, we took turns to guess what the many merchants and shop owners, who stand outside their shops, were chatting to each other about from across the street in loud and ebullient voices.

I carry on past to the centre of this hub of hustle, my legs carrying my sleep-weary bones to the bazaar – a place like none I've seen before.

Tightly packed together are stalls of vibrantly coloured spices in huge cloth sacks. Stalls of fruit and vegetables larger than the largest we'd get back home, of honey or nuts, meat and fish … some smelling more questionable than others but interesting all the same.

The smell of spices, earth, raw meat and countless bodies all merging into a unique blend that can only be found within this shack of tinned roof and plastic sheeting. Outside of the food bazar are tall stands with anything and everything you might need – from electrical goods to shoes, knives to prams.

Today though, I keep inside the food bazaar, occasionally greeting sellers to whom my custom is becoming regular. They've always been kind to me, they could easily take advantage of my ignorance but never do. They seem to enjoy helping and teaching me things. I used to find this place intimidating but now it's quite the opposite.

I pick my way through Gina's list of ingredients, which she left at reception before her run this morning. There's not much, to be fair, but I can feel my arms lagging by my sides as the weight of what she needs from me grows heavier by the moment. The heat of the afternoon sun is sucking the air from around me and is warming the bodies of the people squeezing past me – making me squirm from their clammy touch.

As soon as I get everything on the list I head outside where the air, although not clean like at home, is at least less stifling. I head back towards the new city, where the fancy buildings by the riverside lie and where Eagles Bridge awaits to take me back to the hostel. I stop before I reach the bridge, my body begging for a moment's rest, my legs hollow and my arms aching. I sit on a stone bench, uncaring that the rest of it's been claimed by a couple taking selfies. I lean back against the hard stone, taking a deep lungful of air in an attempt to catch my breath.

Between my sleep being thrown out from doing nightshifts and the loss of my usual training, I can feel my body weakening … I just didn't expect it to happen so quickly.

I know I should take advantage of the pool outside but a part of me is scared to. The last time I went swimming, I was amazed at how the water held me as though welcoming me back. I pushed my hands back and forth around me, the sensation of the water moving through and round my fingers so satisfyingly soothing, the sound of the rippling water as my body disrupted its stillness like music. It was all so perfect but then I lifted my body from its cradling arms and I sank into the depth of myself.

It wasn't that the water had made me feel weightless; it was that it had hid how heavy I'd become.

I watch as a tour guide walks past me with a group of tourists, one of which is staying at the hostel. I smile brightly at her as she makes eye contact with me but she doesn't seem to recognise me. My warm greeting slips from my lips like it had never been there … utterly wasted. I look around at the fancy outer facings of the buildings around me, feeling as false as they are.

I'm not sure how long I sit on the bench, watching people bustle about their day, but when I finally make it back to the hostel, I pause in the lobby, annoyed that another guest has taken my cubby hole, when I hear my name being called by Gina.

'Hi,' I reply. 'I'm just taking my shoes off.'

I dump them into the box next to the one which was mine before heading into the sitting room.

'Hey …' I come to such an abrupt halt that my body lurches.

A face I know too well is beaming at me while my own smile slips from my face like they've stolen it to wear for themselves. My heart feels like its stopped and yet I can feel its shallow pounding within my chest.

'Stephen,' I say breathlessly, like the air's being knocked from my lungs.

'Surprise,' he says eagerly, getting to his feet and coming towards me.

I catch sight of Gina's delighted smile, her hands clasped like she's resisting the urge to clap at her own excitement, of Lev and Hale nudging each other and Smarty's giant grin as Stephen embraces me, his arms mercifully hiding me from sight so that no one can see the horror in my eyes.

Chapter Thirty-four

JOY – AGE 25

I sit at the end of the dinner table, my eyes flicking from one enthralled face to another until they settle on Stephen's. His voice is droning on like a distant engine as he tells his tales about our school antics to a captive audience. I watch his lips moving but my mind refuses to pick out their meaning. For each memory of friendship, of laughter and adventure he shares only deepens my sense of repugnance towards him. I wonder, when he runs out of teenage tales, how he'll fill the eight-year gap of his presence.

I look down at my plate, its contents a challenge to consume. I don't feel like I'm really here. I keep thinking the fork in my fingers will fall through them. I quietly put my fork down and grip onto the outside of my thighs, starting a little at the eruption of laughter, my lips automatically lifting into a smile in case anyone glances at me but no one does. I examine their happy smiles, beaming grins, their bodies leaning forward and back almost in slow motion to my eyes with the momentum of their laughter. I catch Stephen's gaze. The smile still planted on my lips but it's harder to hide things from those who were as close as we were. I know he sees it, for his own smile falters and he drops his gaze before glancing round the table at all the empty plates.

'Shall I clear these away?' he offers, getting to his feet.

For the first time since I arrived, I don't rush to help. I watch as Stephen does that for me. Comfortably manoeuvring around the hostel as though he's always been here, chatting and laughing with Hale and Lev like they've known each other for years – it's me who feels like the stranger now.

'What shall we do this evening?' Gina asks.

It takes me a moment to realise she's talking to me.

'Ehh,' I stutter, glancing around the room for inspiration. 'We've not had the movie night we talked about yet.'

'Perfect.' Gina smiles, adding towards those in the kitchen, 'Can someone check to see if we still have popcorn?'

'There's three bags,' Hale replies a moment later.

'I'll start arranging the chairs,' I say quickly, getting up from the table.

I drag the nearby sofas into a semi-circle and arrange the long coffee table to be at the centre. I do a quick headcount before pushing an extra couch in behind the first row.

'Joy, can you put these on the table?' Hale asks as I finish up, holding out the divvied-up bowls of popcorn for me to take.

'Sure,' I say, reluctantly going to the kitchen to take them.

I numbly put the bowls on the coffee table and turn back around, staggering back a step as I nearly collide into Stephen and the bowls of popcorn he's balancing in his arms.

'That was close. Sorry,' he laughs.

'S-ok,' I stutter, moving around him.

A memory of him, from when we were fifteen, flashes across my mind so swiftly I can barely hold onto it, but I hear the ghosts of laughter whisper in my ear. I used to play my memories like a beloved film. I know each one so well that I don't need to see it to know how Stephen will struggle to balance four overfull glasses of iced tea, how his expression will alter as he trips on something which isn't even there. I can almost feel the ice cubes and the chill of the tea as it drenches Logan, Amy and I while we lie on the grass basking in the sunshine. The shock, the hysterics, the decision to leap into the loch with our sticky clothes still on because what was the point in removing them?

'Anyone got any more food?' Lev asks.

'I-I have some crisps,' I tell him, dazedly.

'I have some wine,' a guest offers, as Lev nods his approval of both.

'I have chocolate,' Lev offers.

I add my large bags of crisps to the mound, astounded by the treasure trove of goodies people have procured from their rucksacks and suitcases. I slowly head to the kitchen to help Hale make hot chocolate with honey and cinnamon – my recipe now a hostel favourite.

I set the cups on the worktop; watching as Stephen and Lev muck about by throwing bits of popcorn into the air and seeing who can catch it with their mouths. I close my eyes to an image of Logan dropkicking a bag of crisps. The pop as the bag bursts and splinters of crisp explode from the bag like shrapnel. The shock on Logan's face and the laughter which ensued. I open my eyes as Stephen's laughter outdoes the memory of it. It always came so effortlessly to him.

'You ready?' Hale asks, nudging me affectionately with her elbow, her hands occupied by the teapot of hot chocolate.

I follow her into to the communal room and sit on the corner of the couch at the back, perched up on cushions so I can see over the heads of those on the couch in front of me. Glad that the lights Smarty extinguishes shield my face – I don't think I could hide the gulf behind my eyes much longer.

From the glow of the TV screen, my gaze is drawn to Stephen. It's as if my eyes are trying to convince my brain of what it knows is true but what it wants to deny. I watch as he laughs in time with everyone else to the comedy on show; even the Turkish girl who speaks no English laughs to be a part of the reaction. My fingers itch to reach out and touch the back of his head just to see if he's solid.

'I promise I'll be here for you.' He had assured me, when I first became ill, with such conviction that I never doubted it couldn't be true.

Instead, I watch the clock. When I estimate that there's only half an hour left of the film, I bid everyone goodnight. Hale and Smarty protest but I'm unwavering. I tell them I want to be up early. I tell them I still have to call home, I tell them what they want to hear to make it acceptable to them … the recovering sick are experts at it. We make our needs fit into your wants. Our explanations must suit your expectation. We are the sick masquerading as the healthy. We compromise ourselves to make ourselves acceptable to you. We all do it … it's just some are more proficient at it than others.

I quickly get ready for bed, my legs feeling laboured as I drag them into the dorm and up into my bunk. I wrap the blankets around me, wishing they were arms to hold me in the darkness – I can barely recall the feeling. A memory of being squished tightly inside a cold tent, the same night as the ice tea drenching, dances across the dark ceiling.

After a while I hear footsteps, the creak of the door being opened. The drip of light becomes a puddle.

'Joy, are you awake?' Stephen asks quietly.

I know I should answer, I know it's the right thing to do, but I can't find the words to speak. Instead, I listen as he rummages around in his bag, using the light from his phone to guide his way. Then, he disappears. When he returns, a little while later, he does so with Hale. The sound of whispered voices asking questions, of zips being undone, the rustle of bags being rummaged in gently filling the void of stillness. The soft shhhh-ing noise of the curtains being drawn around beds like a gentle calling to sleep. Eventually the creak of the metal bunks, as each individual gets comfy, settles down into silence.

I resist for as long as I can, but eventually I pull back my curtain slightly to look down upon Stephen's bunk. The glow from the world outside illuminating his features enough to see his closed eyes through the gap in his curtains.

I have so many questions but I'm not sure I can bear the answers.

When I wake the next morning, I automatically pull the thin blanket over my head, resentful of the light. I sigh, wiping at my damp eyes, memories from yesterday slowly clicking into the emotions. Stephen ... how I long to wake up and be the fun-loving girl in his stories. The one who was so alive, so full of freedom and feeling. She was damaged, we all are, but she was unbroken. I'm tired of waking up with eyes which weep in the night.

With a second sigh, I throw off my blanket and begin to get sorted for the day.

I head downstairs but the place is conspicuously empty. I follow the sound of voices and music to the back garden. Pausing, I take in the people milling around the outdoor table, which has been set up for breakfast, a speaker on the windowsill playing an upbeat song in a foreign language.

'You're up at last. We were going to get you,' Lev says, as I appear in the doorway.

'This looks impressive,' I say, squinting to see the bowls of fresh fruit, pancakes, the pot of porridge, tubs of cereal, fresh bread and pastries against the bright morning light.

'Stephen reminded me that we've been neglecting how lucky we are to have such nice weather,' Gina tells me, setting out cups full of cutlery. 'He was saying how you always eat outside when it's sunny because you get so little sunshine.'

'Yeah, that's right,' I say, glancing at Stephen as we take our places around the table.

'So, we went out and got some breakfast things. I forgot how nice it is to do this. Thank you for reminding us, Stephen,' Gina says warmly, forever inclusive.

Unthinkingly, I take the tub of cereal being handed to me and swiftly pass it on in exchange for the bowl of porridge and fruit.

'You want the pancakes and the chocolate spread over?' Stephen asks me.

'No, thanks,' I say.

'But they're your favourite!'

I shrug. He's not wrong, he's just ignorant as to why I can't eat them. Another note of his absence.

'Oh, Joy, I meant to say, we're getting a new coffee machine. When it arrives can you set it up and show us how to work it?' Gina asks enthusiastically.

I freeze, my stomach dropping. '… Sure, erm, only it probably won't be the same as the one we had back home,' I say, quickly spooning a mouthful of porridge into my mouth in the hope that Gina will discontinue the conversation.

'I'm sure you'll still know more than me,' Gina says generously, but her kindness only sends a chill down my spine. 'It'll be so nice to have a barista here!'

I flash her a smile, deliberately not looking at Stephen as his quizzical eyes land on me – burning my skin as harshly as the intense sun above us. I stare down at my porridge, my stomach clenched tightly, as I shift uncomfortably in my seat.

'Joy, I was thinking as well, it might be nice for you to show Stephen and the other new guest round the city – like what Hale did when you first arrived?'

'Sure,' I say, wrapping an arm around my waist to catch my swooping stomach.

Chapter Thirty-five

JOY – AGE 25

Stupid things sick people say and do to other sick people:

- It's not a competition, people, and yet ... it is! Look, we don't have much to boast about so being able to stand in a room and go, 'Well, I'm sicker than you are,' is the equivalent of a healthy person going, 'Well, I got 90 per cent in my exam and you only got 20 per cent.' It's pathetic but that's life.

- 'Ugh, I'm on twenty-three tablets a day.' – Congratulations, come back to me when you're on eighty a day and then we can talk.

- 'Today's a special day, I have an extra five tablets to take on top of my twenty-three.' – Well I'm still on eighty but, if you want, I can talk you through all the other shit I have to do to survive?

- 'You're looking so well.' – Shame on you! You should know not to judge someone's health by how they look.

- 'I've got a two-year treatment plan. It's so arduous.' – Yeah, well mine's lifelong so sod off.

- 'I've been ill for two months now and it's just ruined my life.' – Oh, you're a funny one ... try being ill for a decade or more then come back to complain about it.

- 'The public hospital is taking ages to treat me.' – Boo hoo! You're getting seen by the best specialist, you're getting all the medical support, financial support, moral support they have and not paying a thing for it. You want to know what I got … NOTHING! I was told my illness was inside my head and literally left to die.
- 'I'm just constantly on edge not knowing what's going to come at me next.' – Oh please, your condition is clean cut! You either get your life back or you die at the end of your treatment … I have to spend my life not knowing when I'll achieve either.

I ponder the question, friend or foe, enemy or ally, while we wander the new city, our bodies occasionally bashing against the other as we navigate the busy streets. I pause now and then to point out statues Hale had shown me and to tell the stories behind them to Stephen and the other guest.

'In my city, we have statues twice that size,' the guest remarks scathingly.

I resist the urge to roll my eyes at what will be his fourth comment like this. I'm quickly coming to the conclusion that my initial reaction to him was correct … he's a twat. I've nicknamed him the hair-merger because all his facial hair grows into each other – so that he only has a small sliver, where his eyes and nose are, that's hairless. I find nicknames easier to remember than actual names, even if I can't use all of them out loud.

We meander towards the old city, the bustle of life growing more intense in the constricted streets. I try to keep an eye out so that I don't lose either of them but I'd be lying if I said I'd be upset if I did. We pause to look in some of the shop windows. The hair-merger taking an excessively long time pawing at the glass of the jewellers, the extravagant gold necklaces and rings with huge rubies and sapphires reflected in his greedy eyes.

'These are so flimsy. Back home we have necklaces that are so strong it's impossible to break the chain,' the hair-merger says.

'Let's hope no one tries to strangle you with one, then,' I say before I can stop myself, both of us turning to Stephen as he coughs on the sip of water he's just taken from his bottle. 'You ok?'

'Yup,' he says, wiping his mouth with the back of his hand, a grin on his face as he looks at me.

I eagerly head towards the bazaar. 'This is where we get most of our fruit and veg,' I tell them, as the tin roof comes into view.

I take another four or five strides towards it before I notice that the hair-merger isn't beside us anymore. I pause to look around, only to find him looking at the bazaar with revulsion.

'I'm not going in there,' he says.

I glance to Stephen, trying to assess his reaction and therefore what mine should be, but his face is uselessly blank.

'The tour guides back home take us …'

'I'm not a tour guide,' I say with a dismissive shrug.

He stares at me, seemingly unsure of how to react. His long hair beginning to stick in clumps to his head as the afternoon sun intensifies.

'Why don't we meet you back here,' Stephen quickly steps in to break up the mini standoff. 'In, say … an hour.'

'I think I'll walk on my own,' he says curtly.

'Ok,' I say, turning to Stephen to see if he's ready to continue. 'What?'

'Nothing,' he says quickly, while the hair-merger disappears into the crowd. 'You're just … ehh, a bit more direct these days. I'm just not used to … It's not a bad thing. You were always feisty. I mean—'

'After you,' I instruct Stephen dryly, cutting him off before he covers his grave with topsoil.

One down, one to go, I tell myself as we head into the narrow passages of the outer labyrinth of the bazaar.

I thought Stephen might have been hesitant in here, like I was when I first came but, of course, he takes it all annoyingly in his stride. Confidently navigating and dodging out the way of oncoming people on a mission to get their desires.

'Should we get some grapes and we can sit somewhere and eat them?' Stephen suggests, pointing to the stall to the left of us which is full of fat purple grapes.

'Ehh, sure,' I say, with little enthusiasm but unopposed to the sugar boost.

With our grapes in a paper bag, we head up to the only place I had left on my mini tour. We don't speak much as we walk alongside the twisting road, which leads up to the castle.

I'm glad for the silence, despite the awkwardness that lingers within it. Walking up the hill is trying enough for my lungs without the added exertion of conversation.

'Look at that,' I say, pausing to point to a cart being pulled by a mule while a fancy estate car nips impatiently at its back. The old and the new, the poor and the rich, compressed together.

With Stephen's eyes upon it, I take the opportunity to gulp at the heavy air, my legs humming more than I'd like them to. I snap my mouth shut and give a smile that feels more like a grimace as he looks around to see my reaction before turning back to the cart. I stretch my neck from side to side, as he watches the slow procession, feeling the sharp crunching and popping at each rotation of my neck. Beads of sweat prickling my skin. Most days the heat is pleasantly warm, but today the intensity of the sun is making my body heady with heaviness. Once the cart passes us, we continue back up the hill to the car park where tour buses have hijacked most of the available spaces.

We take our time going through the crowded gates. Two security guards sit to one side playing cards – not even pretending to pay attention to the coming and goings.

'Everyone stares at you here,' Stephen remarks, glancing self-consciously about us.

'You get used to it,' I tell him, as we pass into the main fort.

From outside, the fort looks complete but inside all that's left, protruding from the grass, are the skeletons of buildings.

'What's over there?' Stephen asks, looking at a modern building to the left of us.

'It was the museum but it's closed down. The government couldn't afford to staff it apparently.'

We wander round the remains of the old buildings before heading to a set of stairs which takes you up to the wall. The castle, when it's quiet, closely rivals the bazaar as my favourite place to go.

We meander along the wall walk, pausing now and then to wait as people take pictures. After a while, the number of people thin as we get to a section where the wall slowly disappears into the ground; until there's no wall at all and only the uneven and crumbling slabs of the stone walkway that still exist at our feet. Back home this would be sectioned off with high metal railings and plastered with warning signs, but here they like to weed out the smart from the stupid by leaving it untouched. I lower myself onto the edge of the stone, the weight of my legs dangling gloriously over the fort's wall, the deep drop of stonework ending in a steep entangled embankment followed on by another road.

'Are we allowed to sit here?' Stephen asks, looking around for some sign or warning as I did when I first came here.

'They don't care,' I tell him.

He cautiously lowers himself down beside me, the bag of grapes between us like a separation barrier. He pulls a stem of grapes off the stalk and hands it to me before doing the same for himself. We sit amidst the noise of car engines and horns, of the chatter of tourists and of children screaming gleefully as they play on the grass behind us.

'So … you're a barista,' he says, neither as a question or a statement.

I glance at him before looking away. I can tell he wants to tell me off for lying but we both know he holds no moral standing between us.

I pick at the empty stem from which I plucked the last grape off just minutes before, the sweet juices still pungent in my mouth. I watch Stephen covertly from the corner of my eye. It would be so tantalisingly easy to go back, to be the friends that we once were to each other, but I'm trapped between wanting his friendship and mistrusting it. It was one thing to act the dance of civility and even friendship back home, to use his presence to help me reunite and meet new people. It wasn't hard to act like there was no hurt feelings between us even though we both knew there were. I look back out towards the city. I was safe back then, safe in the knowledge that I didn't need anyone to survive. And it's true, I don't need anyone, but it's also a lie. We all need someone; it's built into us to crave company and connection. I just can't trust his.

I can feel him watching me, hesitant to speak and clearly eager to. I don't know how to respond to him being here. I can hardly continue the standoff I feel towards him though but I suspect neither of us wants to face the questions and the hurt which lies between us. When I finally look at him, his gaze isn't focused on me at all but on Logan's watch. Unthinkingly, I cup it with my other hand as though to protect it.

'What are you going to do when this machine arrives?' he asks, finally breaking the silence.

'I'll figure it out,' I shrug.

'Why did you tell them that in the first place?'

I look at him, trying to discern if there's scorn in his voice. 'All I said was that I worked in a café ... which isn't a lie,' I point out.

'Wait ... you mean the one you worked in when you were fifteen? That was ten years ago,' he says incredulously.

'It still counts and it's still not a lie,' I say, throwing a bruised grape from inside the bag down into the abyss between my toes.

'Just a huge stretching of the truth.'

'More a stretching of the timeline,' I say, unable to resist a small smile at what I see as a victory over him.

He shakes his head, reciprocating my smile begrudgingly.

'Why are you here?' I ask, my voice so small it's almost smothered by the laughter of children.

'Gina messaged me, maybe a week or so after you arrived, to see if I wanted to come out. She said she thought it would be nice if I could come, what with ... so you were still here with a friend.' Stephen pulls the last grape off his stem and throws it away. 'Apparently, all three of us were meant to come but she already had two TravelerStay's booked so she could only take two of us.'

I nod. It was neither the answer to the question nor the

answer I was looking for, but maybe, for now, it'll do.

Once the bag of grapes is half demolished, we head back to the hostel. Stephen puts the rest of the grapes into a bowl and leaves them for people to pick at.

'How was it?' Gina asks, when she sees we've returned albeit minus one.

'Good, although we lost the other guy,' I say, filling her in on what happened.

I'm surprised but relieved when she doesn't seem particularly bothered. She's probably seen his type hundreds of times before. Still, I'm glad to learn that the hair-merger has yet to return.

I head into the back garden to find Hale, Lev and three other guests in the pool; throwing a ball back and forth over a net that they've pulled across the centre.

'You coming in?' Stephen asks, coming up behind me, having done a speedy change into trunks.

I follow him outside, watching as he jumps into the pool, the water jumping up and showering out around him. Hale splashes him as he surfaces with a grin. Tentatively, I take off my socks and sit on the edge, my burning feet soothed by the cool water, which massages them as I swirl my legs back and forth and around.

'Just come in,' Hale calls to me in frustration.

I stare down at the water, my eyes transfixed by the light dancing on its surface, the rest of my body envious of the relief my legs are obtaining – my mind longing to join in the laughter.

I get to my feet, stumbling a little until I find my stride as I head inside. Within a few minutes, I'm back outside in my bikini. I set the timer on my phone to ten minutes and leave it by the table.

'Yes, get in here,' Hale calls elatedly, when she spots me heading towards them.

'Joy is on my team,' Lev chips in quickly.

'Lev, you can't keep switching teams,' Hale puts back, as I slowly ease myself down the steps.

As Lev and Hale bicker, my muscles sigh in the blissfully cool water which cradles my body. I lift my feet for a moment and allow myself to float. Once I'm certain I won't sink, I let my head tip back, the water lapping at my ears and distorting the sound of the praise and commiseration of the game beside me. I can't believe I let fear hold me back in allowing myself to feel this free.

'Joy, I need your help to beat them,' Hale calls impatiently.

I let my feet sink to the tiled ground, using it to push myself forward through the water, as I swim under the net to her side of the pool. My limbs move cumbersomely, unused to the motion.

To say that I'm a hinderance more than a help to Hale, the guest and Stephen (who took Lev's place when he abandoned ship after seeing how useless I am at catching) would be an understatement. Stephen even took to standing behind me, to catch the throws I missed.

'Is that someone's phone?' another guest asks.

'What?' I call, out of breath.

'Someone's phone's ringing,' she repeats.

'Oh, that's mine. Thanks.'

Reluctantly, I pull myself out of the water. I hesitate as my legs adjust to taking my weight. They feel wobbly but they hold me steadfast. I turn my alarm off and sit on one of the loungers.

'You not coming back in?' Stephen asks.

'You're useless but we need you,' Hale calls.

'I'm good here for now,' I tell them, content to watch because at least I got to take part.

Chapter Thirty-six

JOY – AGE 25

Over the following week, being in the pool becomes a part of our routine. The water has always been Stephen's second home and, with his enthusiasm for it, we all naturally migrate towards it. I've been carefully building it up, though, from ten minutes in the pool and thirty minutes out, into being able to spend twenty. I know it doesn't sound like much but given the amount of walking we do each day exploring and how I'm feeling … I'll take any victory. They all think my breaks on the lounger are for the vanity of getting a tan … I don't disillusion them.

'Even he is not as pale as you and you come from the same place,' Lev tells me, comparing Stephen, who happens to be standing beside me.

I shrug. I'm just glad that my skin's no longer so translucent you can see the veins in my face.

Stephen and I often do strokes together while Hale, Lev and whichever guests are around muck about in the other half, Stephen's arms and legs gliding through the water with only the slightest of ripples while I splash and slap the water like a horrified cat.

'You'll get it back, though,' he tells me.

'Yeah,' I mutter, out of breath and clinging to the edge of the pool while he pushes off for another lap.

I watch him glide through the water, my eyes lingering on the smooth ripples he creates. There's something hypnotic about water. It holds a fine line between pleasure and danger. I watch my arms sway in the current of those around me, the image neither clear nor distorted. I used to spend so much time in the water. I adored the suppleness of it, how it sounded, the feeling of it moving around me. All those hours Logan and I spent helping Stephen train at the weekends. Both of us racing alongside each other or me timing their laps. So much time spent in the echo of the pool. The shouting of the crowd calling on those in the water during race day. I never competed like Stephen. I didn't have parents who could afford it or had the time to take me to training the way he did.

I let myself sink until my nose is barely above the water, the sun glistening off the surface dazzling me. Slowly my head slips beneath the water, the sounds above the surface warped, my body swaying in the current of their movement. I sink lower, daring myself to see how long I can stay there. I sense something coming at me but before I can open my eyes it hits me; the water subduing the blow to my ribs but still knocking the air from my lungs. I emerge, gasping in air and water at the same time, frantically looking around to see what hit me and coughing as I choke on the water I've inhaled.

'You ok? I didn't see you,' Stephen asks in alarm, grabbing my arm to keep me above the water.

'Yeah,' I stutter, rubbing my ribs.

'You trying to drown yourself?' he jokes.

'… I'm going to head in,' I tell him, ignoring his comment.

With my towel wrapped tightly around me, I hasten inside.

'Joy,' Gina calls as I race pass the kitchen, my damp feet slipping slightly as I stop. 'Lev's leaving the day after tomorrow and he's really keen to see Polsa before he goes. I thought it might be nice for a group of us to go tomorrow, if you want to come?'

'He's leaving?' My hand freezes in its attempts to catch the droplets from my hair.

'He's decided it's time to move on,' Gina tells me, pulling a bowl from the cupboard below her.

I watch her with dismay. Lev always seemed like a permanent feature; I never considered him leaving.

'Yeah, that sounds nice,' I say defeatedly. 'What all's there?'

'There's not much there really but it's beautiful. I was thinking we could get the boat across to the old monastery and have a picnic at the ruins. It's just a quick walk up the hill.'

'How big is the hill?' I ask, my mind whirls to prepare an excuse.

'It's not a long walk. Maybe an hour.'

She lied! That's all I think to myself, as I pause on the path to try and inhale some air, gazing up at the steep mountainside masquerading as a hill while the rest continue up the path with the gusto of gazelles.

'An hour my ass,' I mutter, the gap between me and everyone else growing by the moment.

I sigh in the air, which feels starved of oxygen – my legs pleading for a break. One step, one breath, I tell myself over and over again. Forcing my feet to move in time to my mantra.

'You ok?' Hale calls down to me through the trees, directly above me, on the winding path which constantly curves back on itself.

'Yeah ... I- I just dropped my phone so had to go back for it,' I lie. Why break the tradition of fabrication? 'I'll catch up, it's ok, keep going.'

I hate myself for saying it because the last thing I want is to be alone, I don't want to be the only one struggling or who finds this hard. I keep my head down, watching my feet as though concealing how far I have to go will make it easier. I spin Logan's watch round and around my wrist as I walk, the metal back sticking to my warm skin. Slowly, I look up as the path starts to curve, resigned to the potential prospect of sitting on a rock until they decide it's time to go home, only Stephen's already sitting in the spot I'd earmarked as mine.

'Hey,' I say, coming to a stop beside him, my voice shockingly breathless.

'Hey,' he says, shifting over on the rock to make space for me.

I take a deep breath and glance out to the dark water in the ravine before us. The humming in my legs and the cringing in my lower back, though, force me to concede to sitting beside him. Without saying anything, he hands me the water bottle in his hands.

'Thanks,' I say quietly, taking a gulp from its open mouth.

I don't ask why he's sitting here; I already know and I both hate and admire him for it. It was things like this that made us friends in the first place.

'You ok down there?' Gina calls.

'We're just taking in the view,' Stephen calls up to them.

I look down at the loose stone path at my feet, my eyes swimming in all the things I'm trying to escape.

'Take your time,' Gina calls back, sounding pleased by our appreciation of the place.

I can feel Stephen watching me but I'm afraid to look up, to let him see me crumble. I examine my pale legs, which reveal nothing of the pin pricks which hollow them out with every step I take each day, and the arms which show nothing of the screaming pain within them. I am the perfect contradiction of strength and weakness, beast and beauty, living and dying, and I don't know how to reconcile with any of them.

'You want to go back?' Stephen asks.

I shake my head without thinking. There is no going back, that's the whole reason I'm here.

'I just need another minute. I'll be fine once I've had lunch,' I tell him, to abate the voice which whispers a warning that I might get there but that doesn't mean I'll get back.

I can do this, I tell myself, cupping the watch on my wrist. I can do anything ... I bite the inside of my mouth, wanting to weep as the untruth of it hits me.

We sit in silence, Stephen showing no signs of impatience as we wait until I decide my body has recovered enough to go a bit further. Stephen automatically walks ahead of me. Dictating the slow but steady pace we take. He pauses at each curve in the path and, without saying a thing, he waits until I've regained my breath before continuing.

Eventually, we make it to the top. On the edge of the rockface are wooden huts on stilts, their red-tiled roofs sticking out against a backdrop of grey rock and the green vegetation around it. I spot Gina at the one furthest away. The open sides and rickety floor look like another Maltdonian test between human bravery and stupidity. The ground here slowly rises up to where the ruins of the monastery sit at the peak of the slope, the stones of the square building slowly eroding and crumbling. The decorative tower at its centre is miraculously still standing; the tiles on the roof jumbled together and bowing downwards, like crooked teeth, from where the stones and beams have fallen beneath them. I gaze around me as my breathing eases and steadies. It's breathtaking, only for once it's in a good way, like something out of a film. I spent so many years in that sofa bed, trapped in that room, watching images like this one on TV and wondering if such places really existed.

'Logan would like it here,' Stephen says, coming to stand beside me.

'Yeah, he would have,' I say gently. '... You know the mountain you can see from my bedroom?'

'Yeah.'

'Logan and I were going to climb them in the summer.'

He nods, a small smile lifting his lips.

'Like old times,' he says.

'Like old times,' I repeat.

We look at each other; with so much to say and no words to say them with, I walk away.

Chapter Thirty-seven

JOY – AGE 25

I was right about feeling a bit better after eating. The salami and chicken pick and mix, along with the sweetness of the fruit after and the long rest to observe the view, revived a lot of the energy I'd lost. We sat in the hut, the flimsy wooden railing the only thing before us and the drop into the ravine below. Standing at its ridge like we were on the edge of the world. We watched as the sun sets in a shifting array of splendid red, orange and gold – each of us content enough in the other's company to simply watch the beauty before us.

The moment the sun sunk out of sight, Gina suggested we head back before the darkness settled in. The walk back was strenuous but the loose and slippery path, which constantly shifted underfoot, meant that it was a slow descent for us all and not just for me.

When we get back to the city, we slowly wander back to the hostel, a sense of calm amongst us which is stolen as we enter the hostel into the clamour of newcomers. Shoes litter the floor and rucksacks wrestle to consume the lobby.

'That'll be the group we were expecting,' Gina comments, picking her way across the lobby to the communal room to help Marty.

I step aside to let her past while the rest of us take our shoes off.

'You're the one who stole my cubby hole,' I state, watching Stephen freeze as he puts his trainers in the hole I marked as mine on my first day.

'You're the one who keeps stealing it whenever I go out?' he remarks, turning to look at me.

'Possibly,' I admit reluctantly.

'There's heaps of spare ones,' he points out, gesturing to all the options open to me.

'You should tell them that,' Hale says, shoving her shoes into a random cubby and nodding towards the group, who are mulling noisily around the reception.

We edge our way around them and head to the shelter of the kitchen but none of us have any notion to cook.

'Shall we get a takeaway in?' Hale calls to Gina.

'Yes, go ahead,' Gina agrees, glancing up distractedly from the computer screen.

Hale pulls out some menus from the drawer and spreads them out on the worktop.

'Pick what you want. These ones are the better restaurants though,' she says, singling out four options for Indian, Chinese, Mexican and Turkish.

'I've never had Turkish before,' I remark.

'Seriously?' Hale says. 'That's sorted, then. Pick what you fancy and let me know.'

I survey the menu, trying to discern what I'm able to eat from the scant descriptions versus the price of the dish. I pick Tavuk Basti without any real idea of what it is before heading up to the dorm to put my head down until it arrives.

I'm barely in my bunk, though, when Gina opens the door.

'Sorry, Joy, I didn't know you were there. You're going to be sharing the room for a few days. Do you know which bunks are taken?'

'These ones here are empty,' I say, pointing out the free ones.

'Thanks,' she says distractedly, leaving me to it.

Minutes later, the door is opened and Gina proceeds to show the girls their bunk. I inwardly groan as I pull my headphones from the shelf above me and connect it to my phone, trying to drown out their loud chatter, in an unknown language, as they clatter about the place.

When I'm called down for dinner, I find most of our group from today are sitting outside under the canopy outside, their bodies framed around the fire pit, which is slowly flickering into life, the flames almost dancing to the Latvian music playing in the background.

'This one's yours, Joy,' Hale tells me, handing me a plate. 'Although Lev nicked some so feel free to steal some of his.'

'I was just checking it,' he says with false sincerity.

'That's ok,' I smile, sitting next to one of the Portuguese guests.

'Wine,' Stephen offers.

'… Sure,' I say hesitantly, taking the glass he's offering to me.

'How is it?' Hale asks, halfway through our meal.

'It's good,' I say nodding my appreciation. 'You want to try some?'

'Yes,' Lev says slyly, leaning eagerly over.

'Here, help yourself,' I laugh, holding my plate out to anyone who wants to try a bit, each of us giving and taking from the other under the fading light and the growing glow of the fire.

'Those people who arrived are playing at the volleyball tournament over the weekend. We should go,' Hale suggests.

'That would be fun,' I agree, taking a mouthful of rice.

'You should enter,' Hale mocks.

'I would be a brilliant team member,' I shoot back, pointing my fork at her to emphasise my point.

'Maybe as a ball collector,' Stephen mocks.

'I have many skills,' I retort.

'What are they?' Lev asks curiously.

I purse my lips ... thinking. 'I can belly dance.'

'What,' Stephen exclaims. 'Since when?'

'Since always.'

'Show us, we need proof,' Hale calls excitedly, nudging me to get up.

'I'll teach you,' I compromise.

Hale leaps to her feet, Lev following behind her, while Stephen turns up the music.

'Come on, all of you,' I say to the other guests, getting them up in a line.

'Right,' I say, trying to remember what to do before exclaiming, 'Ok, for a chest roll, all you do is draw a diamond shape with your chest. So ... push your chest up to the sky then over to the left, down to the ground and then over to your right and up again. And just build it up until you can do it faster.'

'I need much bigger chest,' Lev laughs, clasping his pecs.

'What are you up to?' Gina calls curiously, from the back door.

'Belly dancing,' Hale replies happily.

'Looks fun but I'm afraid you need to turn the music down soon. It's almost ten.'

'Course, sorry,' Stephen says, hastening to turn it back down.

'We should go to the park and finish these off,' Hale suggests eagerly, holding up her glass of wine.

'I'm not sure that's a good idea?' Steven whispers to me as he passes me some of the glasses he's collected off the ground from dinner.

I know he's right. I just want, for one night, to be like everyone else. I turn to Hale, opening my mouth ready to say no but smile instead.

Ten minutes later, we find ourselves wandering along the park's path. In the daylight, the hedges which are cut with precision into people and animals come to life. The huge sculpture of a boat made out of flowers stands out against the green of the grass and the tall trees but here, in the darkness, you'd never know they were there. At night, the only thing we can see is the winding path, illuminated by lamps, weaving majestically into the darkness.

We stop at the bandstand to sit on the benches and play music, the wine diminishing as the laughter develops.

'What music is this?' Lev asks, as a song which sounds like it's come from a musical comes on.

'Oh, I don't know,' Stephen says, rushing to change it.

'No, no, I like it,' Lev says, getting to his feet and holding his hand out to me.

I eye it hesitantly for a moment before taking it and giving a small curtsy, smiling as he spins me under his arm like Logan did at Kate's party – I stumble as the world keep twirling long after I stop but Lev's hand keeps me balanced.

I try to copy Lev's feet as he tries to waltz with me, his voice loud in my ear as he sings along as best as he can.

I glance around as Lev and I dance about the bandstand; Hale and Stephen are dancing away while the other two guests sit watching with bemusement. I lead Lev over to the start of the bench, which runs along the length of the bandstand, and use his hand to steady myself as I step up onto it. I skip around it as Lev extravagantly dances a Russian dance below me, one hand extended to the air for balance and the other held onto mine, the two guests leaping to their feet to get out the way. When we get to the end, Lev grabs my waist to lift me down, his grip tight on my waist as he lifts me up over his head. I soar over him for a moment before there's a rush of air, a swooping, a falling. I'm like a stunned bird against a window.

'Joy, you ok?' Stephen's panicked voice fills my ear from far away and then up close.

The rush of feeling as my body, at first numb, reacts to the shock of my landing.

'Ouch,' I cry, bursting out laughing as I lie on the ground, my legs still entangled in Lev's arms.

I slowly sit up and look at my elbow. Tentatively, I touch it, the dark mark and stinging of the deep graze making me laugh further.

'You've scarred me,' I laugh hysterically, consumed with giggles, which I know are irrational but feel so freeing that I let them devour me anyway.

'We are joined for life! We have same scar,' Lev holds up his bloodied elbow to compare against mine.

I can't stop giggling as I allow him to heave me to my feet and guide me to the bench. I watch, with eyes that smile at their joy, as they dance around the bandstand. The two guests slowly coming out of themselves and tentatively joining in, with increasing enthusiasm that's in sync with the increasing depletion of wine. I feel like a teenager, illegally drinking in the park and doing nothing other than being foolish and fun. Not a thought to anything other than what's happening right here and now. No consequences, no considerations, no fears. I am simply … free.

Chapter Thirty-eight

JOY – AGE 25

The tops things the recovering sick don't say for fear you wouldn't understand

- Just because we look like we can function normally now, it doesn't mean we do ... we just have coping strategies that make it appear that way.
- We might walk and talk and act like everyone else now ... but we function at a pain level which could cripple most. Everything we do we do despite the pain and exhaustion inside us.
- We push ourselves to the extreme just so we can do what you do so easily.
- When you're not around we unravel, disintegrate and are pushed back into the shell of our disease because we're so exhausted and sore from trying to function in a society that is so inhospitable and unthinking towards us.

I listen as time passes, the passing of each song counting the minutes that I lie in the darkness of night, unable to sleep. I take my headphones out, the music unable to relax my body. Sleep should come easily after our day at the monastery and our drunken wander of the city but the dorm feels too full with the new guests. The sound of so many bodies breathing out of sync with each other is a drone my tinnitus has readily taken up. The hostel has never been this busy since I arrived. Strange how the energy here constantly changes and shifts like the ebb and flow of the ocean as new people come and the old go. I can feel the hostel's energy pulsating, too full and lively for sleep. My legs twitch and jump under the thin sheet that covers me, my nerves shooting and dancing with sparks that have me wanting to cry out in pain.

In desperation, I throw my sheet off and clamber down the ladder of my bunk, almost falling as I misplace my feet. As quickly and quietly as I can, I head out of the dorm and down the stairs, the movement helping to release some of the pain. I go to the bathroom just for an excuse to be moving about so late. I pace in the small space of the bathroom, the cool tiles blissful to the burning heat in my body. I want to lie on the tiles, absorb their coolness, but instead I run my wrists under the cold water until my hands go numb and I can't feel my wrists.

Reluctantly, I resign myself to having to go back to my bunk and wait it out.

Come morning, I clamber down from my bunk, my head swaying a little as I get to the bottom. I lean forwards, holding onto the bar of the ladder to keep me steady until it passes. I just need food, I tell myself, straightening up. I head downstairs, my every step a groggy effort.

'Morning,' Smarty calls cheerily from reception.

'Morning,' I say, my smile an effort to reciprocate.

I briefly smile hi to Claire, who's sitting at the table having breakfast, before sticking the kettle on – squeezing past Hale and Lev to get to the cups.

'Good morning,' Lev calls eagerly, holding out his arms for a hug.

'Morning. You excited to leave?' I say, stepping into him.

'Yes and no.'

'Where are you going?' I ask, still hugging him.

'To where someone will take me,' he says, giving me a little squeeze.

'You're hitchhiking?'

'Yes.'

'You're not worried it's dangerous?' I ask, growing increasingly aware of how uncomfortably hot it is today.

'No,' he says, drawing out the word. 'That is how I got here.'

He gives me a squeeze before letting me go. I resume making myself a cup of tea and one for Stephen, who's sitting on the couch looking at one of the books from reception. I carry them into the communal room, my body swaying, and the world swirling, my mind deserted with distortion. I try to put the cups on the counter but miss. They clatter to the ground but I don't see them smashing as I fall …

'Joy, Joy, can you hear me?'

I open my eyes, the view before me hazy and undefined.

'Joy?' a woman's voice calm but firm says close to me before adding more distantly, 'give her some space.'

I open my eyes again. I can't tell where I am or who I am.

'Hey.' I try to look at who's spoken but their face blurs again.

'It's Stephen, you fainted. You're ok though.'

'I … I,' my voice comes out at a childlike pitch, innocent and defenceless. I try to sit up but I can't tell which way is up and which is down.

'Try to drink this.'

My hair is tugged and pulled at as a hand is moved under my head and holds it up. I feel the cold rim of a cup and the steam of something warm inside it near my lips. I sip. I am an obedient child. The sweetness of the tea hits my mouth and dances around it.

'That's it. Try another sip or two.'

'That's it. Just another mouthful and you're done,' Aunt Beth said, inserting the straw in my mouth once more, the very effort of swallowing too much for my body to bear.

I try to recoil from the memory but the hand is holding me steadfast. I sip again and again, the people around me coming more clearly into view.

'Do you feel ok to sit up?' Gina asks.

I nod, using my numb limbs to help push myself upright, although the hand at my back does most of the work. I lean forwards as the world inside my head rotates round and round. A hand, too big to be Gina's, rubs circles on my back and instinctually I know it's Stephen.

'Are you nauseous or dizzy?' Logan once asked me, rubbing my back in circles when I took unwell before him. 'Joy?'

Shit, I think, my gut sinking into the floor. I can't bring myself to look up into the unravelling of all I've created here. To see all their worry and concern. I was doing so well. I want to weep for the grief of their disillusionment.

'Eat this,' Lev says, crouching before me and handing me a chocolate bar.

'Thanks,' I say, my voice a meek whisper.

I gingerly take a bite of the chocolate bar, my teeth sinking a little bit into the chocolate before a piece snaps off. It's been years since I had a chocolate bar. It's both delicious and disgusting. The sweet fat turning into a horrible aftertaste but I know it'll help in a way that nothing else can. Stephen helps me onto the couch and I sit for a while as everyone around me slowly drifts off to get on with what they were doing – occasionally throwing me a curious glance or a small smile. I hate it. I hate myself. I can feel myself shrinking and shrivelling up as I sit there.

I have a second sweet cup of tea before tentatively heading back upstairs with Stephen following behind me in case I faint again. I'm glad he can't see my face, for the depth of my mortification can't be hidden. I feel his hands on my waist to steady me as I wobble on the stairs, like Aunt Beth's hands would be when she cleaned me. He waits for me as I pause at the top of the stairs to catch my breath. The darkness inside me deepens with each step I take back into the routine of being someone who's sick. I can still walk, I'm still standing … It's not the same, I tell myself but it doesn't matter, the damage is done.

I don't ask, I just take his bunk instead of attempting to climb into mine; he owes me close to a decade of friendship, I decide his bunk is the least he can do for me.

'You want anything?' he asks awkwardly.

'My phone and headphones,' I say, my voice so feeble it's almost non-existent. 'They're under my pillow.'

'Thanks,' I say, as he hands them to me.

He looks around, unsure of himself.

'You want me to stay for a bit?'

I shake my head, my voice stolen by the hand of dejection.

'Ok, text me if you want anything,' he says, leaving me alone in a world that I don't want to be in.

I spend the afternoon in bed, mostly sleeping and then watching TV on my phone, unable to face the people that await me downstairs. Nature eventually forces my hand though and I reluctantly head downstairs to use the bathroom, pausing on the way back up to watch everyone mucking about in the garden. Someone has gotten their hands on some water pistols and everyone is running about the place chasing after each other, laughing and shrieking with the carefree joy of adults reunited with the child within, their faces alight and eyes wide with life. I sink down onto the stairs to watch them, my mind revelling in the sight while my heart sinks into sadness.

'You can join them, you know,' Smarty says, appearing from the back corridor, making me jump.

'Yeah, maybe,' I say, scanning the garden again. 'Where's Lev?'

'He left,' Smarty tells me, leaning against the bottom of the railing to the stairs.

'He didn't say bye,' I say.

'He didn't want to wake you,' Smarty says.

'But he didn't say bye,' I repeat, glancing out to the garden as it hits me that I'll never see him again.

'People come and go. It's what they do,' he says with a shrug. 'You should never expect people to stay, just enjoy them while you have them.'

I should know that better than anyone … so why doesn't that abate the pain of their departure?

'You feeling better?'

'Yeah, I was just too hot and hadn't had anything to eat. That's all,' I say automatically.

'Of course,' he says, looking at me with an odd expression of understanding and something close to disappointment. 'You coming?' he asks.

I pause, reluctant to break free from the cocoon upstairs

but slowly I nod and together we walk outside. Smarty instantly grabs a discarded jug and fills it up at the pool to throw over anyone who comes near him. I sit on the lounger, watching and occasionally ducking a misaimed shower of water.

'How are you feeling?' Gina asks, perching herself on the lounger next to me, patches of her top damp from the water fight.

'I'm fine. I was just too hot and hadn't eaten,' I reiterate.

Gina pauses as though pondering what to say. 'I understand that you've been ill for a long time now. Maybe tomorrow when you're feeling better, we can have a chat about it. Stephen's offered to do your shift tonight so you can rest,' she says.

I shake my head, my hand wrapping themselves around my stomach and her blanching words.

'I- I can do my shift tonight. I'm fine now I've slept,' I try desperately to assure her. 'I'm fine, honestly. I'd never be able to sleep anyway after sleeping all afternoon.'

She looks around us, the sun rippling across her dark hair, seemingly weighing up her options.

'Ok, if you're sure. It should be quiet tonight. There's the volleyball tournament at the park tonight. I think most of us are planning to go to it and we're fully booked so there'll be no check-ins.'

I nod, relieved at my reprieve. I watch her walk away before my eyes hunt out the only person who could have betrayed me.

I keep to myself as we have dinner, all the while trying not to notice how those who saw me fall are tiptoeing around me, handing me things like I might drop them.

'It's ok, you sit,' Hale says, when I try to help clear up, her words kind but like a shard in my gut.

269

I want to protest but I've lost my standing to do so, so I sit on the couch and sip my tea, now void of sugar, watching as the anticipation in the room grows while my dejection burrows deep inside me.

'Are you sure you don't want me to do your shift?' Stephen asks.

'No, thanks,' I tell him shortly, as Gina calls to everyone that it's time to head out.

'Are you ok?' he asks hesitantly, his body already twisted towards the door.

'I'm fine,' I state, still cradling my empty cup.

'Ok,' he says, sounding rejected.

I watch as everyone slowly files out of the hostel; the hum of their voices dies away like a fading swarm of wasps. I get up and wander about. Gina wasn't lying when she said that most people would be out; the hostel is empty. I stand in the middle of the communal room, lost and alone.

I sit for a while longer before wandering outside in a body which doesn't feel like mine anymore. I slowly gather up the water guns and put them on the bench by the back door - the back light and the fairy lights strung up all over the place illuminating my way. I gather up the towels left forgotten by their owners and take them inside, folding up the ones owned by guests and laying them neatly on the table by reception, with a note asking guests to collect them. I add a smiley face to ensure I sound friendly. I wash the ones which belong to the hostel, tidying and cleaning the external world around me to try to contain my internal one. I add fresh towels to the bathrooms, even though they don't need them. I hunt for anything that's out of place, but I find little.

I try watching a film to fill the void of time but I can't

focus. I stare blankly into the nothingness, overwhelmed by the emptiness inside me. The boredom of a life unfelt draining me of any notion of desire. I turn the TV off, the noise nothing but an irritant, my reflection staring back at me on the dark screen until the person shown in it blurs before my stinging eyes.

I stand up carefully, as though I might break the body which isn't mine. I stare about me, remembering moments which don't seem to belong to me anymore. I try to smile but the weight of my falsehood drags my lips down. I feel nothing. Even the burning pain in my neck and joints doesn't seem to belong to me. I head outside, the bright stars more visible now the back light's off. I wander round and round the pool as though waiting for someone to push me in – to wake me up. I pause at the bottom of the tower to the flying fox, my eyes taking in the tape to stop people going up it. In one swift motion, I rip it off. The weight of my body balanced between my arms and legs as I step up onto the first rung of the ladder. Up and up my body takes me until I reach the top. I lean over the edge of the railing; wondering how far it would take to fall. I ease my body down to sit on the edge where jumpers stand, my legs dangling, staring out at the city lights. I watch people moving around on the busy streets, all these moving dots of people and all these cars. A city full of people and yet no one can hear my scream.

My eyes fall to gaze down into the darkness of the water, the moon and the stars shining up at me. I hold onto your watch as I straighten my legs, my body tipping forwards as I straighten. I release my last breath into the rush of air flowing past me as I fall into the stars.

Chapter Thirty-nine

JOY – AGE 25

My body slams into the water, pain bursting to life, smarting my skin like the fist of a thug as my body plummets to the depths. My feet hit the bottom, shockwaves juddering up from the base of my feet and up my legs as they slide out from under me. I don't fight it. I let myself sink till I lie at the bottom of the peaceful pool, the cold water encasing me. I close my eyes against my lungs, which no longer long for air. I see myself on the sofa bed. *A living corpse … rotting from the inside out. I don't want to die but what is there to make me live?*

'Are you saying this is all in my head?' I asked the doctor.

'Yes.'

Suddenly, I'm trying to pull myself off the couch but my excuse of a body fails me. Trembling, panting, pain shooting up my legs, I fall back onto the couch. Defeated.

I'm on the utility room floor, sobbing from the pain and exhaustion of hanging up a few socks.

Then, I'm outside as snow falls around me, my hesitant feet crunch down onto frostbitten grass. Dog eagerly awaits me.

I'm smiling as Logan twirls me inside the gazebo.

I'm in a club with our old group of friends reformed, we hold hands just in time to count down to the New Year in FIVE, FOUR,

THREE, TWO, ONE ....

'You promise, no matter what happens, you'll go?' Logan's voice whispers to me in the water.

'I promise I'll go ... no matter what!'

'I'm not Joyce,' I cry. My Aunt Beth's face burned into my vision.

Lev's force-feeding me crisps I don't want as we sit on the dorm floor. Smarty's wearing a pillowcase like a nun's habit over his head.

I'm dancing in a bandstand, the glow of the park's light dancing around me as I spin with my arms held wide.

So much pain, so many moments ... so many. I don't want to live in a world as cruel as this one. So why can't I stop fighting? Why can't I give in? Why, despite it all, do I refuse to believe that this is all I can get from this life? I don't want this. I want more. I need more. I want to be alive. I want to live.

I open my eyes, the ghosts of my past floating around me in the dark water. I push up from the tiled bottom, my feet and ankles yelling in agony, my arms pushing at the water around me, my lungs dully burning as my body reclaims its fight for air. I feel like they'll explode and implode at the same time. Sparks dance before my eyes as I keep pushing myself upwards, the moon above me swaying and distorted as I reach out a hand to it.

I look around the dark depths as the water buffets me and something grabs me around my waist. I push and squirm away from its grasp but it holds me fast. My legs kicking into another's as we move upwards until our heads break the water. I gasp for air, my tired body struggling to keep my head above the water, my eyes staring into Stephen's. I look away, coughing as the water catches the back of my throat. Struggling to keep myself afloat, I start to swim to the edge of the pool, my weakened limbs struggling to move me forwards but Stephen's arm still holds me and pulls me alongside him until we reach the side.

I cling onto the edge of the pool, resting my head against it for a moment before pulling myself up onto the edge and clambering out of the water, the weight of my body crushing me as I drag myself backwards until I'm leaning against a nearby lounger. I cough into the night, hungrily hunting for air.

'Are you hurt?' Stephen asks, crouching down and looking me over in the scant light from the back door.

I shake my head, wondering how true that actually is.

'What were you thinking! Why did you jump? What were you trying to do ... Were you trying to hurt yourself?'

'No,' I say, quickly. '... I- I just wanted to feel.'

'What do you mean?' he asks, his eyes boring into me.

I shake my head, trying to clear it, trying to focus over the pounding of my heart, the words desperately slipping out before I can stop them. 'I just, I don't know.'

I look away, unable to meet his gaze in the gulf of silence that ensues. I draw my knees up to my chest, feeling a fool.

'Joy, come on, you must have known how dangerous that was. That water's too shallow to jump from that height. I'm surprised you haven't broken your ankles.'

I look into the worry-filled eyes of the person I would once have done anything for, that I'd have done anything to have back in my life, the friend I don't know how to forgive.

'Why do you care?' I whisper with dejection.

'Joy,' he utters, wounded, his face as etched with shocked as if I'd slapped him.

'Seriously, why do you care? Why are you even here, Stephen?'

He opens his mouth but it takes a moment for him to find his way.

'Because ... I wanted to make things right and I hated the idea of you being here alone.'

'Then why did you tell everyone that I'm sick?' I say, my voice quiet with the betrayal residing in it.

'I had to. Joy, you passed out and wouldn't wake up. Claire told them that she'd seen you taking a load of drugs ... They were going to call an ambulance. They were talking about pumping your stomach.'

I shake my head, not wanting to accept the rationality of his explanation.

'... Maybe I shouldn't have come here,' he finally says in defeat, clasping the back of his neck and leaning back against the opposite lounger. 'I feel like all I've done is make things harder for you.'

'What did you think would happen?' I say in dismay, wrapping my arms around my knees, my muscles tensing against the chill seeping inside of me.

'I don't know. I just thought we could both use a friend. After what happened with Logan, I get how what I did hurt you and ...'

'No,' I cut him off, my voice growing. 'You don't get to compare the two. Logan died; he had no choice. You did, you chose to leave me, you chose to walk away ... I was dying, Stephen, and you left me.'

'I know, I'm sorry, I ...' but words seem to fail him, his entire face seems to sag under the shame of my words.

'You don't even know what you're apologising for,' I tell him bitterly, a cool breeze making me shiver. 'You have no idea. Why ... why did you leave me?' I ask, wiping resentfully at the burning streaks my tears leave on my cheeks.

'I don't know,' he all but whispers, unable to look at me, his head slumped towards the ground so that his face is mostly in the shadows.

'That's not good enough,' I tell him stoically. 'Am I ... am I that easy to walk away from, am I *that* disposable?'

'No, no of course not ... I just, I didn't know how to be around you. I never knew what to say or do or ...'

'No,' I cut him off, my eye so brimmed with tears that I can barely see him. 'That's not it, it can't be it, it's not enough. It's not.'

He runs his hands through his wet hair, standing it up on end before flattening it again.

'I don't know, Joy. I was scared and I was weak and it was too big and it was easier to walk away than it was to stay,' he lists frankly, his voice desperate for me to understand, for him to find a way out into somewhere better. 'You want me to tell you that I felt pathetic because there was nothing I could do to help you. That I didn't know how to be around you. You weren't you anymore! It hurt, Joy, it physically hurt to see you and watch you disappearing and turning into something unrecognisable.'

I look away, unable to stomach his words.

'... How do you think it felt to live it? To lose everything that ever mattered to me,' I say, the words coming out as a whisper which longed to be yelled. 'You got to walk away after visiting me, you got to carry on with your life. I had to live it, I had to fight it every second of every day. I still have to; I will never be free ... It was never your job to heal me, but it *was* your job not to break me.'

'I ... I was young. I was sixteen, Joy.'

'So was I,' I bite back.

'I know, I'm just saying, I'm not that kid anymore. I want to make things right and I want ...'

'... What? You want what, Stephen?' I sigh, exhaustion deflating my resentment, my wet clothes so uncomfortably cold that my skin hurts underneath them.

'We were so close. Friends like you and Logan are rare and I don't want to lose another friendship like that if there's a chance to make it right.'

'I don't ... I don't know how to be your friend, Stephen, I don't know how to be anyone's friend anymore. I- I don't know how to forgive you.'

'I know, I don't know how to forgive me either,' he says quietly.

'You left me,' I say, the full impact of the words sending my world crumbling before me.

'I know,' he repeats, as though acceptance of my words is his only defence. 'I will never forgive myself for leaving you. Staying ... staying just cost more than leaving – at least that's what I thought. I never knew how sick you became until Logan told me at New Year. Joy, I had no idea. I should have been there for you and I'm sorry.'

I hold my breath, trying to contain the gut-wrenching sobs that want to burst from me. So much pain that just can't be contained, that can't be let loose. Out of everyone who left me, Stephen's departure was the worst. I know it's not fair to hold him to a different standard to the rest, but out of everyone ... I never foresaw him forsaking me. I trusted him. I trusted the promises he made me and when I was lying alone in the darkness, in indescribable pain, his promise was all I had to hold onto.

I take a shuddering breath and slowly tip my head back slightly, staring up at the sky and wishing that I was a part of it – tears falling silently down the side of my face, the stars swimming in the ocean of my eyes. I'm so tired of fighting. Of feeling attacked. I'm tired of living in the darkness of the unknown. A fugitive trying to outrun my captor. I want to give in, just once, to something. I want the illusion that someone cares, not because they have to but because they choose to, that I can count on something or someone when I can't count on myself.

'I don't know how to do this,' I say, my confession breaking the little that's left whole inside me. 'I don't know how to live anymore.'

'I know, I know,' he says, moving over to sit beside me, wrapping his arms around me while I openly weep before him, his warm skin and soaking top a strange mixture of comfort and discontent to my shaking body, as I sob for the life I lost and for the friend who held me together.

'Breathe, just breathe,' he whispers gently, rocking me from side to side.

I gasp for snippets of air; my lungs feeling frozen. Eventually though, exhaustion stems the flow of my sorrow. My breathing evens and heart slows.

'You're shivering. Come on, let's go inside,' he says, getting stiffly to his feet before helping me up. 'You sure your ankles are ok?'

I nod, my legs raw and tender, my joints reprimanding me for the extra injustice of their lashing.

I head to the bathroom to shower and warm up while Stephen keeps an eye on things – with everything that's happened I forgot I was meant to be on shift. I stand under the warm water, my body shaking violently, the stringing heat slowly expelling my internal chill. When I get back downstairs, Stephen's sitting on the couch under a blanket with two steaming mugs on the table before him. He holds the blanket up for me to join him. I hesitate before sitting beside him. While I arrange the blanket around me, he reaches over to get the mugs and we drink them in silence.

'What if they ask me to leave?' I ask faintly, after half an hour.

'Then I'll leave with you,' he says simply.

Chapter Forty

JOY – AGE 25

By the time everyone arrives back after the tournament, tired but elated, Stephen's asleep on the couch next to me. Somehow, despite the bustle, he sleeps through them all gathering together in the communal room with cups of tea and slices of toast, bags of crisps and eager recanting of antics.

'He made it back then,' Hale remarks, looking at Stephen's unconscious form.

'Yeah,' I say into my mug.

'He said he was going back to check on you,' Hale tells me.

'So, it was a good night?' I ask, eager to change the subject back to tonight's adventures.

'Very good, thank you for taking me,' one of the guest's chips in.

'You're welcome,' Gina tells her, perching on the arm of the couch. 'I'm going up. Joy, if Stephen stirs then perhaps suggest that he goes up to bed, but if he doesn't then don't worry. It won't hurt for one night but I don't encourage people to sleep outside the dorm rooms.'

'Course,' I say placidly.

'I'll see you in the morning before your shift ends,' she says to me, her words like a lead weight in my stomach. 'Night everyone. Remember to keep the noise down.'

There's a chorus of softly spoken goodnights as she walks away. Slowly, those that are left start drifting away to their beds too.

'You ok?' Hale asks me, her brows pinched. She is, as always, the last one standing.

'Yeah, think so,' I tell her.

'We should draw on him,' she says mischievously, eying Stephen's unmarred features.

'Or put whipped cream on his hand and tickle his noise,' I suggest.

'I did that once ... turned out they weren't asleep and I ended up wearing the cream. Anyway, goodnight.'

'Night,' I say meekly.

I watch her until she disappears round the corner before getting up to turn all the lights off – bar the lamp at reception. A calm sense of stillness settling over the hostel as the last of those still awake finally fall asleep. I lie on the couch nearest reception, my body shivering in the gloom, under a mound of blankets, waiting for my body heat to build within the fabric.

'Come here,' Stephen's groggy voice comes from the other couch.

I sit up sluggishly, wondering if he's talking in his sleep but his arm's holding up the blanket he's under.

'I can hear your teeth chattering from here.'

I hesitate.

'Hurry up, I'm making a draught.'

I stand up on unstable legs and join him in the warmth. He pulls the blankets around me. It's like stepping into a warm house after being out in the cold. He wraps his arm around me as my body shivers and shakes. I smile sadly, remembering, before

I got ill, us all camping as teenagers and being squished together in the tent like Stephen and I are now. I slowly relax, my body gradually shaking less and less. For once I give in. I stop fighting. I let myself be held when I can't hold myself.

I lie on the couch and watch the early morning light shift and transform as the sun sets, not wanting to move from the warmth of another beside me. Eventually, I sit up, my body recoiling from the coolness of the room. I drag my lethargic form to the kitchen to make a pot of tea.

'Morning,' Gina says brightly, from across the bar top, as I steep the tea.

'Hi,' I say, my hand instantly going to my stomach as it forms loops.

'Can I get some?' she asks, looking at the pot.

I nod and set about making her a mug.

'Would you take it into the back room?'

'Yeah,' I mutter, her smile brief as she turns and walks away from me.

I take a deep breath as I pick up our mugs and carry them into the back room, glancing surreptitiously at Stephen's sleeping form as I pass.

'Thanks,' Gina says, taking the mug I hold out for her. 'Have a seat.'

I do as I'm bade, sitting on the only other seat available, my hands cupping my mug for comfort.

'How are you? You gave us quite a scare yesterday.'

'I know, I'm sorry,' I say, stealing Stephen's line.

'Stephen explained to us that you have a long-term illness, Lyme disease, is that right?' she says, the word sticking in the air like a swear word said at church – dirtying the sanctity of somewhere sacred.

I nod, my throat too constricted to form words.

'I did some reading on it last night but is there anything in particular you think I should know about your condition?' she asks cautiously.

'… No, I don't think so,' I say, my voice stronger than I expected it to be.

Gina pauses as though about to ask something but the humane hand of caution holds her back, as she considers me for a moment longer, before forging forwards.

'… Why didn't you tell us? I checked yesterday, there was nothing on your TravelerStay form.'

'Would you have taken me if I had?' I ask plainly.

She ponders this for a moment, her eyes holding my gaze.

'No,' she says, looking away and sitting back for a moment before looking back at me. 'No, I wouldn't have, and that would have been my mistake because you have done everything asked of you … more, in fact. Far more than those who don't have your limitations.'

Gina pauses, her eyes fixing on something to the left of me. I follow her gaze to the newly delivered and still boxed-up coffee machine.

'I'm guessing you're not a barista?'

'I worked in a coffee shop before I got ill but no, I'm not a barista. Would … would you like me to leave?' I say, freely offering her my departure to save her from doing so.

'No, not if you don't want to, but Joy, if I may,' Gina says, leaning forwards, 'can I ask that you don't hide your illness. I'm not suggesting that you have to speak about it to anyone but I don't want you to feel like you have to hide yourself here. We don't expect you to be anything more than who you are, so if you're tired and don't feel like taking guests out then you can say that. Or if we ask how you are, you can tell us the truth ... heaven knows, Hale's not shy in telling us her complaints.'

I glance around the room as though searching for a clue on how to reply because, in truth, such a concept feels alien to me. I've spent so many years hiding how I feel for fear of hurting those close to me or for fear of them leaving, but maybe she's right. Why does everyone else have the right to be heard except me?

'We want you to be able to be you and your illness is a part of that.'

'My illness isn't who I am,' I tell her staunchly.

'No, it's not all of who you are but it is a big part of you. I fully understand the desire but denying and rejecting a part of yourself ... it only means that you're at war with it,' Gina tells me, her head tipped to one side as she speaks. I watch the shifting of emotions passing through her eyes, their depth etched with their own understanding. 'I think you will be happier if you find a way to accept your illness.'

'I don't want to accept it,' I say quickly, recoiling in my seat. 'That would be giving into it.'

'Acceptance doesn't mean you stop fighting it ... it just means you stop punishing yourself for something that's not your fault. It means letting the old you go and embracing the new one rather than fighting for something that's gone. From what Stephen told us, you're probably going to have this illness for the rest of your life,' Gina says softly. 'That's a long time to be at war.'

I look away from her, my thumb rubbing at Logan's watch strap, that pip of pain back in my throat.

'It hurts to learn the things that are important in life, Joy, and you've had to learn a lot of those and sometimes in that process you have to let pieces of yourself die to let your new self be born. Your life isn't going to be the same as everyone's, you'll have to do thing differently sometimes and at different times maybe, but if you can find a way to be at peace with that, you won't have to hold yourself to the standards or pace of everyone else. You've been here a month now and it's clear that you care about people and you want to be around them. But you're holding back this huge and remarkable part of yourself and you can only let people in if you're willing to make yourself vulnerable to them. I'm not saying it'll be easy or that everyone will accept you but you need to accept yourself before you'll be able to find those who do … I know I'm greatly overstepping here but I care about everyone who stays here and I want everyone who leaves here to be happier than when they arrived.'

I stare down at the long thin hand ticking on Logan's watch. All I can think is that I never knew it was waterproof.

'I thought you were going to ask me to leave,' I confess, when the silence becomes awkward.

'I'm not thrilled you *hid* your illness but I understand why. The remarkable thing about a hostel is that everyone here has a story, we're a melting pot of the lost, the hurting, the lonely and adventurous. We each have our scars and we each have our own journey. Hostels teach you a lot and you being here has taught me a lot. I don't share the same story as you, Joy, but I know what it feels like to have something hurt you so deeply that it removes you from yourself. You might not know it yet or for a long time to come, but you'll find your way. I promise.'

When I arrived two months seemed like years but, when the turn of the month came, I felt the quickening of time racing down to the day of my departure. I feel like a lifetime here will never be enough but as I gather up my belongings, in preparation for leaving tomorrow, I also know that it's time.

'You ready?' Stephen asks, standing in the doorway to our dorm.

'Yeah,' I say with contentment, getting up and following him downstairs.

I lean against the kitchen counter as everyone mingles about me, a small smile on my lips. It took me a while to realise that the feeling in my stomach wasn't nausea or anxiety but excitement. The entire city is abuzz tonight for the festival of light. The hostel is crammed and humming with anticipation.

I gasp as someone grabs me from behind, lifts me up and spins me around.

'Hello,' Smarty says, lowering me down.

'Hi,' I reply brightly, gripping onto his arms to steady myself as he puts me down. 'Oh, I'm all dizzy now.'

'Sorry – but only a little,' he says. 'Let's go! Let's go!'

He chivvies our group out of the hostel and down the road towards the main street where the festival is being held.

We stop off at almost every stall and drink stand, the streets growing busier the closer we get to the hub of the main event. We slowly make our way to the park, which has been transformed into a wonderland of light, to watch the displays and listen to the local bands playing. For a while we attempt to dance to a mixture of modern and traditional Maltdonian dances but somehow, instead of improving, we only manage to get progressively worse at each attempt. Once we've seen what we want to see there, we head to the main street to wander along the stalls and try an array of dishes … some more appealing than others. The noise and bustle of the crowded streets, which are usually oppressed and polluted by cars, are converted into an upliftingly and infectiously joyous place of excitement, movement, smells and tastes. My neck constantly turning to look about me, my eyes unable to take in all the wonderous sites I see. My senses of smell, touch, sounds and sight are bombarded in a way that elates rather than deflates me.

'We need to go now if we're to see the main acts,' Smarty shouts over the noise of the crowd around us.

I nod and pass on the message to Hale, who's distracted by a group of people walking through the crowd on stilts. Together we head to the main square, where a huge stage has been erected. Already the square is overflowing with people but Smarty's large bulk forges a path for us to get closer to the front. I smile when I feel Hale's hand clasping mine as we follow closely behind Smarty, Marty and Stephen.

'Is this what a festival back home is like?' I ask Stephen, when Smarty decides this will be our spot.

'What?' he calls, leaning towards me to hear me while I check my musician's earplugs are in snuggly enough.

'Is this what a festival back home is like?'

'Yeah, mostly,' he shouts back as everyone erupts into cheers and hoots, whistles and yells.

I look to the big screens to see the band coming onto the stage and picking up their instruments. I can't understand a word of what's being said and eventually sung but I don't care … I'm carried away on the chanting, the smiles and the laughter, the sway of the crowd bumping into those next to them, on the dancing and the moments of affection shared between others hugging and reuniting and living and the fact that I get to be a part of it. I catch Stephen's eye and can't help but smile – the warmth of if spreading inside me. Sometimes, in moments like this, I wonder if everything I went through was all for this single feeling ... of something good.

Chapter Forty-one

JOY – EIGHTEEN MONTHS LATER

*I take my hat off to you, a worthy contender you have turned out to
be, but there are many things you have yet to see.*

*We'll call it a day, for a day and no more. We're both out of
breath so we'll spar no more.*

*Though rest assured, while you think I've gone away … I'm
summoning an army to destroy your day.*

*Silly child, you don't see what I see. You look fixed from the
outside but from the inside I see.*

*I see all the damage that's been done from our war and,
although I know you know it's there, you only feel and never see it
laid bare.*

*While you gamble away, I invite others to play. Infections and
diseases of names unknown. I take them in under my wing and
show them their home. I watch while they feast on the damage I've
done and when the time is right I'll join in the fun.*

For your destruction is of my construction.

*As you go through each day, I am the shadow you can't shake
away. You fight and you fight and I respect your might, but I will
never stop to retain your life.*

*I bow to you, my unexpected foe, I thought you'd be easy to claim
as my own. Your body is my throne and your mind my crown but for*

you, my worthy contender, I'm willing to share a little of both. I was made in darkness by hands playing god, Lyme disease is my name and to their horror they've learned I can never be tamed.

I pull into the car park, pausing momentarily as I pick a spot nearest the office building. Carefully, I reverse into the space. After double checking I've remembered to put the handbrake on, I pause to collect myself. I get out of my little blue car, my pride and joy, affectionately looking at her before turning around and stepping up onto the path which will lead me indoors. If I can live abroad, work abroad, pass my driving test and pass my first university module with distinction then I can manage this, I remind myself forcefully.

I open the heavy door into the building and report to reception. I'm instructed to sit on one of the plush blue chairs nearby, my hand clasped to the outside of my thighs as I nervously wait. I feel my phone's gentle buzz in my bag and when I take it out there's a message.

Stephen: Good luck on your job interview, you'll smash it … as Logan would say. We still on for climbing the mountain tomorrow?

Me: Thanks, just waiting to go in! Definitely, can't wait.

I smile as I put my phone away, before cupping your watch, glad that tomorrow I'll be completing the last of our promises.

'Joy Jack?' a man asks, looking around reception.

'Yes,' I say brightly, getting up steadily to my feet.

'You're here for the part-time position is that right?'

'Yes, that's right.'

'We're ready for you.'

I take a deep breath, smiling excitedly, and follow him in.

A lot can change in a moment, a lot can change in a month and the month after I arrived home, I relapsed. I caught the flu off a friend who thought nothing of seeing me despite being sick herself. I knew within two hours of her leaving my company that I'd caught what she had but I never expected it to cause such damage – it took eight months to regain the ground I lost.

I cancelled the course I had applied to do, too weak to even think of attempting it. Instead, once my health had stabilised, I signed up to do an online part-time degree. It's possibly been one of the best choices of my life. Yes, it might take me longer and it might not be achieved in the conventional manner but I'm doing it and that counts for more than not doing it at all. My life now contains more than just my illness and that's an escape that's turned out to be priceless.

We forever tell ourselves that something wonderful is waiting for us at the end of this great battle to live, to survive, that our comeuppance for life is surely done but that's a lie; it's an illusion we tell ourselves to try and justify what we put ourselves through each day to survive this disease. I won't lie, things don't get easier but they do get better. I will never be free of this disease and the hardship it inflicts upon me every day but I've stopped fighting to reclaim a life that's unobtainable. There is no back, no pause, there is only now. Deep down I've always known that but I was never able to accept it. This is not the life I wanted, nor the one I expected, and I will forever wonder what might have been. This is the life I have though and I've learned that my only job in this world is to find and keep … my Joy.